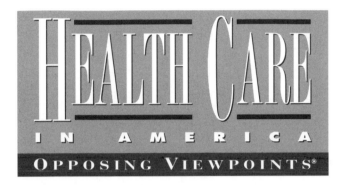

Other Books of Related Interest in the Opposing Viewpoints Series:

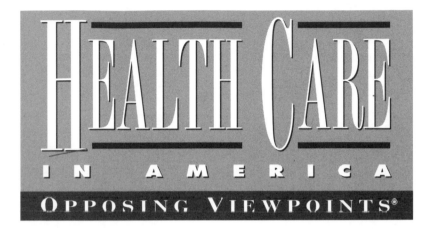

HEALTH CARE
IN AMERICA

OPPOSING VIEWPOINTS®

David Bender & Bruno Leone, *Series Editors*

Carol Wekesser, *Book Editor*

OPPOSING
VIEWPOINTS
SERIES®

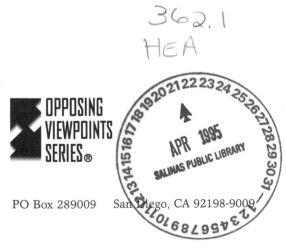

Greenhaven Press, Inc.   PO Box 289009   San Diego, CA 92198-9009

Cover photo: © Rocky Thies

Library of Congress Cataloging-in-Publication Data

Health care in America : opposing viewpoints / Carol Wekesser, book editor.
      p.   cm. — (Opposing viewpoints series)
    Includes bibliographical references and index.
    ISBN 1-56510-135-9 (acid-free paper) — ISBN 1-56510-134-0 (acid-free paper : pbk.)
    1. Medical care—United States. 2. Health care reform—United States. [1. Medical care. 2. Insurance, Health.] I. Wekesser, Carol, 1963–   . II. Series: Opposing viewpoints series (Unnumbered)
RA395.A3H399 1994
362.1'0973—dc20   93-30963
                                                        CIP
                                                           AC

"Congress shall make no law . . . abridging the freedom of speech, or of the press."

First Amendment to the U.S. Constitution

The basic foundation of our democracy is the first amendment guarantee of freedom of expression. The Opposing Viewpoints Series is dedicated to the concept of this basic freedom and the idea that it is more important to practice it than to enshrine it.

Contents

Chapter 5: Would Increased Regulation Improve the Health Care System?

Why Consider Opposing Viewpoints?

"The only way in which a human being can make some approach to knowing the whole of a subject is by hearing what can be said about it by persons of every variety of opinion and studying all modes in which it can be looked at by every character of mind. No wise man ever acquired his wisdom in any mode but this."

John Stuart Mill

In our media-intensive culture it is not difficult to find differing opinions. Thousands of newspapers and magazines and dozens of radio and television talk shows resound with differing points of view. The difficulty lies in deciding which opinion to agree with and which "experts" seem the most credible. The more inundated we become with differing opinions and claims, the more essential it is to hone critical reading and thinking skills to evaluate these ideas. Opposing Viewpoints books address this problem directly by presenting stimulating debates that can be used to enhance and teach these skills. The varied opinions contained in each book examine many different aspects of a single issue. While examining these conveniently edited opposing views, readers can develop critical thinking skills such as the ability to compare and contrast authors' credibility, facts, argumentation styles, use of persuasive techniques, and other stylistic tools. In short, the Opposing Viewpoints Series is an ideal way to attain the higher-level thinking and reading skills so essential in a culture of diverse and contradictory opinions.

In addition to providing a tool for critical thinking, Opposing Viewpoints books challenge readers to question their own strongly held opinions and assumptions. Most people form their opinions on the basis of upbringing, peer pressure, and personal, cultural, or professional bias. By reading carefully balanced opposing views, readers must directly confront new ideas as well as the opinions of those with whom they disagree. This is not to simplistically argue that everyone who reads opposing views will—or should—change his or her opinion. Instead, the series enhances readers' depth of understanding of their own views by encouraging confrontation with opposing ideas. Careful examination of others' views can lead to the readers' understanding of the logical inconsistencies in their own opinions, perspective on why they hold an opinion, and the consideration of the possibility that their opinion requires further evaluation.

Evaluating Other Opinions

To ensure that this type of examination occurs, Opposing Viewpoints books present all types of opinions. Prominent spokespeople on different sides of each issue as well as well-known professionals from many disciplines challenge the reader. An additional goal of the series is to provide a forum for other, less known, or even unpopular viewpoints. The opinion of an ordinary person who has had to make the decision to cut off life support from a terminally ill relative, for example, may be just as valuable and provide just as much insight as a medical ethicist's professional opinion. The editors have two additional purposes in including these less known views. One, the editors encourage readers to respect others' opinions—even when not enhanced by professional credibility. It is only by reading or listening to and objectively evaluating others' ideas that one can determine whether they are worthy of consideration. Two, the inclusion of such viewpoints encourages the important critical thinking skill of objectively evaluating an author's credentials and bias. This evaluation will illuminate an author's reasons for taking a particular stance on an issue and will aid in readers' evaluation of the author's ideas.

As series editors of the Opposing Viewpoints Series, it is our hope that these books will give readers a deeper understanding of the issues debated and an appreciation of the complexity of even seemingly simple issues when good and honest people disagree. This awareness is particularly important in a democratic society such as ours in which people enter into public debate to determine the common good. Those with whom one disagrees should not be regarded as enemies but rather as people whose views deserve careful examination and may shed light on one's own.

Thomas Jefferson once said that "difference of opinion leads to inquiry, and inquiry to truth." Jefferson, a broadly educated man, argued that "if a nation expects to be ignorant and free . . . it expects what never was and never will be." As individuals and as a nation, it is imperative that we consider the opinions of others and examine them with skill and discernment. The Opposing Viewpoints Series is intended to help readers achieve this goal.

David L. Bender & Bruno Leone,
Series Editors

Introduction

"The health of the people is really the foundation upon which all their happiness and all their powers as a state depend."

Benjamin Disraeli, July 24, 1877

The United States boasts the most advanced medical care in the world. American physicians routinely transplant organs and create babies in test tubes and are more successful at treating cancer and other serious illnesses than physicians in any other nation. Wealthy foreigners often seek treatment in the United States, knowing that they will receive the best medicine money can buy.

Most Americans receive adequate, even excellent, health care in this system. These are the insured Americans—those whose companies provide health care benefits or those who can afford private health care policies. These citizens often receive preventive care through regular examinations and they feel confident that, should they become seriously ill, they will be treated and the bulk of the costs will be covered by insurance.

Unfortunately, more than thirty-seven million Americans remain uninsured. They may be employees of the one-fourth of companies that do not provide health care coverage. They may be uninsurable because of a previous medical condition. Or they may be unemployed and too poor to afford private health insurance but not poor enough to qualify for government assistance.

Most of the uninsured cannot afford preventive care such as physical examinations and treatment for minor illnesses. And when their untreated minor illnesses develop into major ones, many of these Americans seek treatment in hospital emergency rooms, where the care may be good but the cost is extremely high for the hospital. When patients cannot pay for this care, hospitals either absorb the cost or it gets passed on to other, paying patients in the form of higher insurance premiums, hospital room rates, and physicians' fees. Some hospitals have even begun turning away uninsured patients to avoid the cost of treating them.

This is the plight of the uninsured. But even insured Americans are not guaranteed complete financial coverage of their medical treatment. Many, when faced with a severe illness, find that their insurance is inadequate or that their insurance company is no longer willing to insure them. For example, eight-year-old Marisa Harvey of Leucadia, California, has only one kidney, which does not fully function. After doctors discovered her problem when she was three, her family's insurance company began doubling their health insurance premium every year. After five years, the family was paying $16,000 annually in health care premiums. They couldn't afford the price hikes and lost their insurance.

Situations like the Harveys' were once unusual, but now are becoming more common. This is largely because many insurance companies are changing their business practices: To compete with other companies for customers, companies increasingly are separating the healthy from the sick, and offering the healthy lower premiums. The sick, meanwhile, face soaring rates and reduced coverage. Because of these changes, thousands of Americans, suffering under the expense of treating a serious illness or paying exorbitantly high premiums, have been financially devastated. And the healthy face the prospect of high premiums should they become sick. As Norman Daniels, a medical ethicist at Tufts University in Medford, Massachusetts, warns, "No one in this country with private health insurance coverage . . . is free from the kind of uncertainty that competition is producing."

Millions of Americans are affected by the gaps in America's health care coverage. But fixing these gaps alone will not solve the nation's health care problems. America must also address rising health care costs and the fact that the overall price the nation pays for health care is already the highest in the world.

In 1991, the United States spent $2,668 per person on health care. Germany, France, Sweden, Italy, Japan, and Great Britain each spent less than $1,700. In 1965, health care costs in the United States were 5.9 percent of the nation's gross domestic product (GDP). By 1991, the figure had soared to 13.2 percent. No other industrialized country spends more than 10 percent. Federal estimates project that if the system is not reformed, by the year 2000 America will be spending close to 20 percent of its GDP on health care.

Excessive spending on health care burdens the nation's economy by siphoning money and resources away from other problems that call for attention. It also impedes economic growth. As former governor of Colorado Richard Lamm states, "The fastest-growing part of any state budget is health. It's an economic cancer that's interfering with whatever else we do in government."

Nearly all Americans agree that escalating health care costs must be controlled, but they disagree on how to control them. A variety of plans have been proposed, from minor reforms to the revamping of the entire system. President Bill Clinton in September 1993 proposed a plan that he believed would guarantee health insurance coverage for all Americans while controlling costs and providing good health care. His critics lambasted the plan, arguing that it was too complicated and would be prohibitively expensive. "The Clinton plan may simply recreate the current mess—too much coverage and too much care for most Americans, too little or none for a sizeable minority, with insecurity and soaring costs for all," argued Harris Meyer, a columnist for *American Medical News*.

Whether they support or oppose Clinton's health care policies, most Americans would agree with his assessment of the health care system as "too uncertain and too expensive, too bureaucratic and too wasteful. It has too much fraud and too much greed." *Health Care in America: Opposing Viewpoints* presents a variety of opinions on why the health care system is "too uncertain and too expensive," and how best to reform it. The book includes the following chapters: Is America's Health Care System in Crisis? Have Physicians Hurt America's Health Care System? Is Alternative Medicine Safe? How Should the United States Reform Its Health Care System? Would Increased Regulation Improve the Health Care System? America's health care system is vast and complex, as are its problems. *Health Care in America: Opposing Viewpoints* aims to address these problems and offer some possible solutions.

Is America's Health Care System in Crisis?

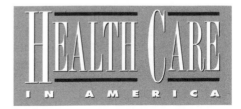

Chapter Preface

Almost all Americans are in some way involved in health care: Patients use it, physicians provide it, insurance companies pay for it, and the government regulates it. Consequently, all have a vested interest in the optimal functioning of the health care system. The problem is that few are willing to accept blame for its problems or change their own behavior to reform it.

Joseph Califano, secretary of health, education, and welfare in the Carter administration, effectively describes this situation:

> Picture our health-care system as a mountain-climbing team struggling to scale an extremely steep cliff en route to a Mount Everest of quality care for all. The lead climber is our spectacular scientific genius and superb doctors and medical centers. But then come those who have lost their footing. One dangling climber is the hospitals, with their empty beds. Another is technology, swinging loose on the rope, unbridled by considerations of the relationship of cost to benefit. Next come lawyers and judges, dragging the team down with malpractice litigation. Then the enormous load of patient expectations, crying out: Do something, Doctor, up to the limit of my health insurance—and don't hold me responsible for my own health. Finally, comes the politician, pandering to providers, needlessly adding to the cost of care. . . .
>
> It's remarkable that our health-care system is still scaling the cliff. But it cannot hope to reach the heights of quality care for all unless we get all members of the team to do their share.

As Califano suggests, all Americans have an interest in the nation's health care system, and all in some way share the blame for its troubles. In the following chapter, the authors discuss both the extent and the causes of problems in the U.S. health care system.

16

"As long as capitalism remains in existence, poverty, misery and insecurity will continue to undermine the health of young and old alike."

Capitalism Has Caused a Health Care Crisis

Nathan Karp

America's economic system—capitalism—can be blamed for the nation's rising medical costs and inadequate health care, charges Nathan Karp in the following viewpoint. Karp argues that only when the United States abolishes capitalism and replaces it with socialism will America be able to solve its health care problems. Capitalism causes physicians, hospitals, insurance companies, and others involved in the health care system to focus on profit instead of on the well-being of patients, the author maintains. Socialism, he concludes, would shift this focus and guarantee that all Americans would receive adequate health care. Karp writes for *The People*, the newspaper of the Socialist Labor Party.

As you read, consider the following questions:

1. What inadequacies of America's health care system does Karp cite?
2. Why are government programs such as unemployment insurance and Social Security inadequate, in the author's opinion?
3. What contradictions did French Utopian Socialist Charles Fourier find in the capitalist system, according to Karp?

From "Health-Care Reforms Aim to Serve Profit Interests" by Nathan Karp. Reprinted, with permission, from the May 1, 1993, issue of *The People*, official journal of the Socialist Labor Party.

For years, and against the background of skyrocketing costs at every level of the health-care industry, corporate executives (including those in the health-care industry), doctors, politicians (in and out of office), social reformers of every stripe, commentators, columnists and the media generally have been engaged in endless discussion and debate on how to meet, and who should bear, the costs of the health and medical needs of American workers and their families.

Like all capitalist reforms, the programs established to date at the state and federal levels have failed to solve the health-care problem. The millions who are covered by those programs are covered inadequately, while many millions more are not covered at all. Even those health-care insurance programs that are part of the fringe benefits that some workers have been able to establish through their unions or have wrested from their employers are far from adequate. Moreover, many of those employers are curtailing or eliminating health-care coverage for their employees or insisting that their employees pay an ever increasing portion of the cost, in many cases even the total cost. . . .

Conflicting Material Interests

Though there appears to be widespread agreement among the various capitalist groups that health-care reform is needed, that is little reason to conclude that the health plan that finally materializes will meet with their unanimous approval, since they have conflicting material and financial interests. As *Newsweek* observed:

> Most of the big-name groups are making a public show of how much they support reform. The American Medical Association, which for decades has fought government intervention, has adopted the slogan, "A time for new partnership." The Pharmaceutical Manufacturers Association has joined with consumer advocates to urge speedy universal coverage. But once the plan is announced and the groups have some specifics to shoot at, the pleasantries will end. "They say they support 95 percent of what we're for," says a Democratic aide. "But how many millions will they spend to defeat the other 5 percent?"

Newsweek went on to suggest that

> The interest groups hit by the plan will inevitably charge that reform is a code word for less health care than the middle class [sic] is getting under the current system. The right to choose your own doctor could become a rallying cry against a plan that will inevitably restrict choice. The specter of rationing [health-care service] will be invoked. The White House will combat these arguments by creating demons on the other side—greedy doctors and insurance companies. Clinton's defenders will argue that for a large chunk of the population there is no choice under the current system, while rationing is

already dictated by ability to pay.

The specifics of the probable controversies may vary somewhat, but *Newsweek's* projected scenario generally is pretty sound. Of course, the White House won't have to create any "demons" since greedy doctors and insurance companies, as well as greedy drug manufacturers and hospital operators, are readily available under capitalism. The abuses practiced by these entrepreneurs in the medical industry are the logical result of the "free enterprise" system. As for the workers and their families, their health concerns and medical needs will receive no more than the minimal consideration that overall capitalist interests dictate. The workers themselves will have no real input either into the ongoing discussions and debate or the final program.

No Real Change

Like past capitalist reforms, whatever new health-care program the Clinton administration may come up with will attempt to deal with effects, leaving the cause untouched. Moreover, whatever limited positive potential the reform program may have will, as has been the case with past reforms, be quickly undermined by power politics, capitalism's inherent anarchy and bureaucratic inefficiency, and the continued insatiable greed of money-hungry medical practitioners and the voracious profit appetites of drug companies and hospital enterprises.

However, even if all those factors could be minimized the possibilities for a comprehensive workable and effective program that would assure adequate health care for American workers and their families is still wishful thinking. All experience demonstrates that reforms bestowed on the workers by the capitalist state are wholly inadequate for solving the problems they are ostensibly intended to solve.

Unemployment insurance doesn't eliminate the misery and suffering of unemployment, it merely "eases" the majority of unemployed workers into that miserable state and inures them to it.

Social Security doesn't terminate economic want for the majority of those who reach old age, it merely creates the illusion that workers will enjoy financial security in their declining years. The fact is, however, that millions of workers on Social Security today are vegetating in degrading poverty.

By the same token, the health-care programs being considered today will not ensure good health and adequate medical care to workers and their families. Rather it will create another illusion—the illusion that workers and their families will be cared for by a concerned society while in fact they will be humiliated into accepting the frustrations and inadequacies of yet another bureaucratic-ridden reform that leaves the cause untouched.

The fact is that the strongest and most influential advocates of health-care reform are staunch upholders of capitalism, a fact that clearly establishes the correlative fact that their reform proposals are intended primarily to serve the interests of the capitalist class and bolster the capitalist system—the very cause of the problem they profess to wish to eliminate.

© 1993 Peter Hannan. Reprinted with permission.

As for those reform advocates who are morally and genuinely troubled by the deplorable state of health care in this nation, they appear to be incapable of understanding the real nature of the problems they are seeking to alleviate. They fail, or refuse, to realize that there is something inherently and irreparably wrong with a social system that condemns millions, young and old, to suffer deprivations and want in the midst of plenty. They assume that the capitalist system is here to stay regardless of how many insoluble social ills it creates. They persist in that assumption even though those ills steadily grow worse despite all the "relief" measures that have been applied down through the years.

Capitalism is a social system riddled with insane contradictions. As the French Utopian Socialist Charles Fourier observed almost 190 years ago:

> The present social order is a ridiculous mechanism, in which portions of the whole are in conflict and acting against the whole. We see each class in society, desire, from interest, the misfortune of other classes. . . . The lawyer wishes litigations and suits. . . . The physician desires sickness. . . . The undertaker wants burials; monopolists and forestallers want famine to make double or treble the price of grain. The architect and builder want conflagrations that will burn down a hundred houses.

In our present society such contradictions are multiplied many times over.

As long as capitalism remains in existence, poverty, misery and insecurity will continue to undermine the health of young and old alike, regardless of efforts to appease them by relief measures. It is the cause of those evils that must be eliminated. That requires that we stop tinkering with effects and turn our full attention to the job of abolishing the poverty-breeding capitalist system and replacing it with socialism—a society that will ensure peace, plenty and healthful conditions for everyone.

"With health care, as with most else, government is not always the solution, it's often the problem."

Government Intervention Has Hurt America's Health Care

Kelly V. Glenn

In the following viewpoint, Kelly V. Glenn states that U.S. government policies encourage waste in the health care system. Government regulations have increased the amount of time and money Americans must spend on health care related paperwork, says Glenn, and have prevented the system from operating effectively in America's free-market economy. Glenn warns America's leaders against enacting price controls and other measures that would hinder the health care system's efficiency. Glenn is the research director at the Competitive Enterprise Institute, an organization that promotes free enterprise and opposes government intervention in the economy.

As you read, consider the following questions:

1. What prevents the U.S. system of health care from being a competitive market, according to Glenn?
2. How would eliminating government regulations affect insurance prices, according to the author?
3. How might price controls increase the cost of pharmaceuticals, in Glenn's opinion?

From "Hands Off Health Care" by Kelly V. Glenn, *CEI Update*, April 1993. Reprinted with the author's permission.

Hardly a day goes by without a report about how horribly expensive health care is in the United States. In 1965, 6% of the gross domestic product was spent on health care. Now nearly 14% of the U.S. GDP is consumed by health care costs, more than double the percentage in Britain or Japan. U.S. spending on health care could soar to a third of the federal budget by the year 2000. Although these figures are staggering, they ignore a significant part of the problem: governmental interference. The share of income spent by consumers on airline travel also increased nearly two and one-half times from 1965 to 1990, according to Robert D. Reischauer, Director of the Congressional Budget Office. However, we are not concerned that consumers are spending more of their income on air travel nor should we be. In fact, as Reischauer points out, in a wealthy country it is not surprising that consumers prefer to spend large amounts of money on good health care and the ability to travel. Nevertheless, it is true that some medical expenses incurred by Americans are wasteful and unnccessary.

A Lack of Incentive

Although U.S. health care is largely privately owned, the extensive scope and scale of government intervention demonstrates that health care is not provided in a truly competitive marketplace. Many individuals do not pay for their health care directly. This is partly a result of government tax policies which encourage lavish employer-provided health care benefits in lieu of higher wages. According to Michael Tanner of the Georgia Public Policy Foundation, approximately 76 cents of every dollar of health care purchased is paid for by someone other than the consumer. As a result, consumers do not have the incentive to shop for the cheapest health care. The prevalence of third-party payments inevitably results in higher prices.

State governments also increase health care costs through mandated-benefit laws. Mandated-benefit laws require insurance companies to pay for particular medical services ranging from chiropractic care to hairpieces. In the 1970s, there were only 30 state-mandated benefits. Today, that number has increased to nearly 800. The inevitable result is an increase in insurance premiums and health care costs overall. Some estimates claim that as many as 9.3 million people are unable to obtain health insurance as a result of these government policies. The Heartland Institute predicts that eliminating these regulations could result in as much as a 30% reduction in insurance prices.

During the 1970s, in an attempt to decrease the number of small, inefficient hospitals and reduce duplication of services, the federal government forced states to enact certificate-of-need

23

(CON) legislation. CON legislation required permission from the federal government before new hospitals could be constructed, new equipment purchased, or new medical services provided. This sort of legislation diminishes competition by restricting entry and results in higher prices.

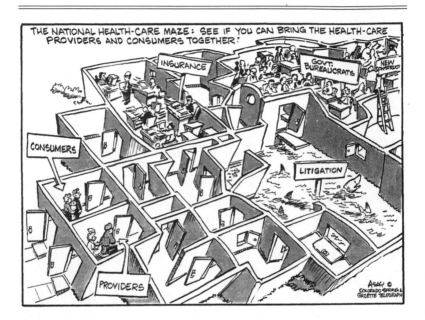

Chuck Asay, by permission of the *Colorado Springs Gazette Telegraph*.

Most of the programs coming from the Clinton administration and members of Congress attempt to contain costs without addressing the underlying cause. Eliminating inefficient regulations would be a good beginning for any overall solution. Also important would be a reassessment of Medicare and Medicaid and the repeal of restrictive occupation licensing laws in the medical profession. Many of the programs which call for increased government involvement, such as price controls and managed competition, would only serve to make matters worse. The price controls imposed in other industries during the 1970s were an abysmal failure. Imposing them today on health care would be no different.

Limiting Drugs Could Increase Prices

Economic consultant Terree Wasley has found that price controls would fail to achieve the intended results and would lead to slower introduction of new pharmaceuticals. Moreover, some relatively expensive medications save the consumer from even more costly hospital stays. For example, the yearly cost of a popular ulcer medication is $1,000, whereas treating an ulcer through surgery costs around $25,000. Limiting the availability of pharmaceuticals through price controls could actually have the perverse effect of increasing health care prices overall.

Perhaps the Clintons should look to their own administration for clues on the feasibility of policy proposals. As Secretary of Energy Hazel O'Leary stated during her confirmation hearings, "I have also learned that heavy-handed Government price regulation does not work." Having worked in the Energy Department under President Carter, her insight comes from direct experience. Her advice should be heeded, for the Clintons will recognize that with health care, as with most else, government is not always the solution, it's often the problem.

> *"The problem of rising health costs is . . . caused by . . . the rapid introduction of valuable and extremely expensive new technology."*

Advances in Medical Technology Are Causing a Crisis

William B. Schwartz

Tremendous advances in medical technology in recent decades have saved thousands of lives. But the expense of these advances is the primary cause of America's rising health care costs, contends William B. Schwartz in the following viewpoint. The author states that only by rationing expensive medical procedures will the United States reduce its health care costs. Schwartz is a professor of medicine at the University of Southern California and co-author of the book *The Painful Prescription: Rationing Hospital Care.*

As you read, consider the following questions:

1. What examples of high-cost medical services does the author give?
2. Why will managed care alone fail to reduce health care costs, in Schwartz's opinion?
3. How would the author ration the use of expensive medical procedures?

Faced with spiraling health care costs, government and business leaders are desperately searching for a solution. Many believe that the magic answer lies in "managed care," a cost-containment strategy designed to eliminate useless care such as unnecessary surgical procedures. The managed-care strategy has great appeal but, unfortunately, it just won't do the job.

The Effect of Technology

The reason is simple. The problem of rising health costs is not caused by the proliferation of useless services but rather by the rapid introduction of valuable and extremely expensive new technology. The unprecedented explosion of medical advances guarantees that the United States will have to turn to rationing if it is serious about reining in costs.

Some Expensive Advances

A few recent examples:

• A new treatment for severe anemia. Nearly all of the 100,000 patients undergoing dialysis for chronic kidney failure suffer from deficiency of erythropoietin, a hormone that stimulates red blood cell production. Its absence leads to severe anemia. The missing substance can now be produced by genetic engineering and is easily administered on a regular basis. Although the therapeutic benefits of the hormone are remarkable, its price tag is daunting: more than $1 billion a year, including use of erythropoietin for the anemia in AIDS patients who take AZT.

• A new kind of pacemaker that prevents sudden death. Some patients with cardiac disease develop rapid, disorganized heart rhythms that frequently cause sudden death. A new device, implanted in the body, can monitor the heart's electrical activity continuously and automatically jolt the heart into a normal rhythm when an episode of electrical chaos occurs. Sudden deaths are virtually eliminated. But given a pool of 100,000 potential candidates and a cost of approximately $50,000 a patient, wide use of the device could impose an annual cost of $5 billion on our health care system.

• A safer material for enhancing the quality of X-ray studies. About 300 deaths a year occur among patients who are injected with a material designed to enhance the quality of X-ray studies of the kidney, heart, brain and other organs. A new material, which costs ten times as much as the old, can wipe out virtually all of these deaths. The added cost: $1 billion a year.

The Revolution of Treatment

The future promises even more rapid and costly progress. In particular, advances in molecular biology and immunology

27

promise to revolutionize the treatment of many serious diseases, from cancer to arthritis. It is hardly a surprise, then, that conventional managed care has no hope of substantially slowing the health cost spiral. In the mid-1980s, managed care and government programs partly offset the upward pressure on costs by reducing the length of hospital stays by nearly 30 percent. But further savings will be hard to achieve because the chief target—unnecessary hospital care—has been largely eliminated by the very successes of the managed-care industry. Even if an additional 10 or 15 percent reduction in hospital stays could be achieved, the effect on the continuing rise in costs would be slight and transient.

How Advances Raise Health Care Costs

For some 50 years, fast-paced changes in technology have been pushing up America's medical costs. According to Joseph Newhouse, a Harvard University economist, health care spending per person grew only 1.4 percent per year between 1929 and 1940 and accounted for 4 percent of GDP [gross domestic product] by the end of that period. After 1940, health care costs grew at an average annual rate of about 4 percent per year and swallowed up 13.4 percent of GDP by 1991. A number of highly technological advances, such as coronary-bypass surgery and hip-replacement operations, have contributed to rising health care costs, but even less expensive therapies have increased expenditures by, paradoxically, keeping people alive longer. For example, the discovery of antibiotics by the 1940s meant that elderly people could now survive a bout of pneumonia only to die of something else like cancer, which is more expensive to treat. And the discovery in the early 1980s of the drug cyclosporine, which prevents the body's immune system from rejecting organ transplants, was instrumental in increasing the number of liver transplants from 15 in 1980 to 3,056 in 1992 at a minimum cost of $200,000 per transplant.

Sara Collins, *U.S. News & World Report*, June 7, 1993.

The choice is clear: We either must pay the staggering bill imposed by new medical technology or we must ration expensive services. Fair and efficient cost control will inevitably require the denial of expensive tests and treatments in cases where costs are high and anticipated benefits small. Serious cost containment will force us, for example, to abandon the use of magnetic resonance imaging in the thousands of patients where there is only a remote chance of finding disease, or under tight budget constraints, admission to the intensive care unit might be denied to the patient who has only a small prospect of survival. Such a focus on "cost-effectiveness" runs counter to most patients' wishes and to the historic ethic of the medical profession. But unless society is willing to accept unchecked increases in health care costs, we will soon face the wrenching choices demanded by rationing.

"Few in Washington are willing to blame what may be the biggest culprit of all: the political influence of special interest groups."

Powerful Health Care Lobbies Hurt American Health Care

Vicki Kemper and Viveca Novak

Many agree that America needs to reform its health care system. Unfortunately, Vicki Kemper and Viveca Novak assert in the following viewpoint, lobbyists for physicians, insurance companies, and others have for years succeeded in impeding reform. The authors write that many of the health care industry lobbies have a great deal of money and power, with which they are able to influence members of Congress. While fighting the lobbies is difficult, the authors conclude that average Americans can succeed in passing health care reform. Kemper is executive editor for *Common Cause Magazine*, a publication of Common Cause, a citizens' action group, and Novak is a staff writer for *The National Journal*.

As you read, consider the following questions:

1. How much have health care political action committees (PACs) contributed to members of Congress? In the authors' opinion, how does this money affect the chances for health care reform?
2. What must happen to motivate Americans to fight the health

From "What's Blocking Health Care Reform?" by Vicki Kemper and Viveca Novak, *Common Cause Magazine*, January-March 1992. Reprinted with permission of *Common Cause Magazine*, 2030 M St. NW, Washington, DC 20036. A one-year subscription is $30.

Opinion polls indicate that 90 percent of Americans believe the nation's health care system needs "fundamental change" or a "complete rebuilding." . . . Proposals calling for everything from minor treatment to major surgery have been pouring out of medical associations, insurance companies, labor unions, businesses, grassroots organizations and ad hoc coalitions. Even the American Medical Association (AMA), which has used money and hardball politics to fight government-sponsored health care programs since the early part of this century, has its own limited prescription for universal coverage. Dozens of reform bills are pending in Congress.

But whether electioneering and political rhetoric will translate into concrete action is another question. Given the obvious need for change, who or what is standing in the way? . . .

Doctors blame lawyers and the government for the current mess. Health care purchasers point to insurance companies that cover only the healthy, while insurers single out greedy doctors and hospitals and unrealistic consumers. Outside analysts frame the problem as a lack of consensus; public interest groups define it as a lack of political courage; and everybody talks about how complicated the issue is.

For all this finger-pointing, few in Washington are willing to blame what may be the biggest culprit of all: the political influence of special interest groups with a vested interest in the status quo. The same insurance companies, doctors, hospitals and drug manufacturers that live off the $700 billion-a-year health care industry are battling comprehensive reform on Capitol Hill and at the White House.

"If the elected officials listen to the public, there are some pretty clear messages," says Stephen McConnell, senior vice president of the Alzheimer's Association. "But if they listen to the organized lobbyists," he adds, "it's a stalemate."

"The people with stakes in the issue who have the most to lose are very well organized, very vocal and very well-heeled," says a high-ranking congressional aide.

What Really Ails Us

Throwing money at the process are more than 200 political action committees—representing everything from the legendary AMA to the obscure Philippine Physicians in America, from the pharmaceutical giant Pfizer to something called the Health Care Committee for Political Responsibility. Together these medical, pharmaceutical and insurance industry PACs contributed more than $60 million to congressional candidates between 1980 and the first half of 1991. PAC contributions from the health care industry have increased far more than gifts from most other special interests: 140 percent during this period, compared with 90

31

percent for all PACs.

Almost half the contributions from the health industry to current members of Congress came from physicians, dentists, nurses and other health professionals; health insurance companies contributed nearly one-third of the total; and the remainder came from pharmaceutical companies, hospitals, nursing homes and other health care providers. The money was carefully targeted: More than $18 million of the contributions went to members of the four congressional committees that have jurisdiction over health-related legislation.

At the beginning of 1992, the top recipients of health-related PAC money all held powerful committee positions: Rep. Pete Stark (D-Calif.), who receives contributions from almost every health-related PAC except the AMA's, is chair of the Ways and Means health subcommittee. Sen. David Durenberger (R-Minn.), a favorite of the hospital lobby, is the ranking Republican on the Senate's Medicare subcommittee. The campaign coffers of Senate Finance Committee Chair Lloyd Bentsen (D-Texas) are brimming with insurance-industry money; doctors and insurance companies are heavy contributors to Sen. Max Baucus (D-Mont.), a high-ranking member of the Finance Committee; and the AMA and other medical associations give generously to Rep. Henry Waxman (D-Calif.), chair of the Energy and Commerce health subcommittee. (Both Stark and Waxman introduced comprehensive reform bills, while Bentsen sponsored a more limited approach.)

Twelve of the 21 senators who received more than $200,000 from medical industry PACs serve on the Finance Committee, which has jurisdiction over Medicare and other health-related matters, as well as tax policy. All of the top 25 House recipients of medical industry PAC money serve in House leadership positions or on the key Ways and Means or Energy and Commerce committees.

Some industry players also distribute so-called "soft money" to the Republican and Democratic parties. In 1991—the first year the Federal Election Commission (FEC) required disclosure of soft money contributions—Aetna, Warner-Lambert, Chubb, the American Dental Association's PAC and the Humana hospital chain each gave $20,000 to the GOP; Blue Cross and Blue Shield gave $29,000 to the Republicans and almost $17,000 to the Democrats; Upjohn gave $25,500 to the Democrats and $23,000 to the GOP; and the pharmaceutical company Glaxo gave $50,000 to the Democrats.

Money Buys Inaction

All that medical industry money hasn't bought better health care—but that's not what it's for. What it has bought is access in

Washington for physicians, hospitals and insurance and pharmaceutical interests, along with inaction on the issue of health care reform.

"We spend our money on those members . . . most interested in maintaining the current system," says Tom Goodwin, public affairs director of the Federation of American Health Systems. The federation, which represents some 1,400 for-profit hospitals, contributed $934,709 to congressional campaigns from 1980 through June 1991, making it the 11th-biggest giver among health-related PACs.

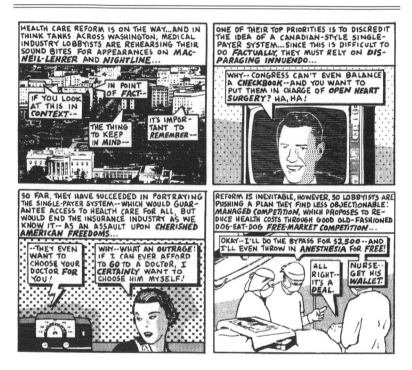

© 1993 Tom Tomorrow. Reprinted with permission.

Like other PACs, those in the medical industry exist to protect their own interests. Consider the primary mission of foot doctors: to make sure that "whatever does transpire, there will be parity and equity for doctors of podiatry," says John Carson, director of governmental affairs for the American Podiatric Medical Association, which has contributed more than $1.1 million to congressional campaigns since 1980. "The PAC has helped us tremendously," Carson says. "I would hate to have been without it for the past almost 20 years."

Or take ophthalmologists, whose primary interests include increased Medicare coverage of cataract surgery and beating back the efforts of optometrists—who also have a very active PAC—to "encroach into their bailiwick." While ophthalmologists make up only 3 percent of the nation's physicians, they are "a very vocal group," acknowledges Cynthia Moran, director of government relations for the American Academy of Ophthalmology. The fourth-largest giver, the academy's PAC has contributed more than $1.9 million to congressional candidates since 1980.

The stream of health-related PAC money into Washington has swelled at a time when U.S. spending on health care has shot past other economic indicators. Health care spending now accounts for 13 percent of the country's GNP [gross national product]—the highest proportion in the world—and it will consume 37 percent by the year 2030 if costs continue to increase at their current rate, according to Richard Darman, [then] director of the Office of Management and Budget.

The average cost of corporate health plans rose 85 percent between 1985 and 1990. Most companies passed along some of the expense to their employees in the form of higher insurance copayments and deductibles. Health care costs have also raised the prices of American-made products. Chrysler says that some $600 of the cost of every car it makes in the United States goes into the nation's health care system. The comparable amount in Germany is $337 and in Japan, $246—one reason why American auto manufacturers support comprehensive change.

Obstacles to Containing Costs

Washington has done little over the years to contain health care costs—at least in part, many believe, because of the PAC contributions that have bought political access for physicians, hospitals and insurance and pharmaceutical firms. "The monied interests have caused gridlock," says Dr. Robert Berenson, a Washington, D.C., physician who served on President Jimmy Carter's domestic policy staff.

Insurance companies represent one huge obstacle. "They are actually against doing anything, because they realize that any kind of reform is going to involve some federal regulation of the insurance industry," says Robert Blendon, chair of the department of health policy and management at the Harvard University School of Public Health.

Most Americans dislike insurance companies, but few politicians are willing to take the industry on. Insurance PACs have contributed $19 million to congressional candidates since 1980, and seven of the top 20 medical industry PACs are affiliated with insurance companies or associations. The National Association of Life Underwriters ranks second, with $5.5 million in contributions to congressional races since 1980. The group's counsel, David Hebert, says candidates who support comprehensive reform are less likely to get its PAC dollars.

Insurance companies such as Prudential, Metropolitan and Travelers, along with the small-business community and a number of health care providers, helped launch a powerful anti-reform coalition, the Healthcare Equity Action League, or HEAL. "We are willing to support . . . incremental, market-oriented changes" that leave the current system essentially intact, says John Motley, co-chair of HEAL's legislative committee and a lobbyist with the National Federation of Independent Business. In an effort to influence the "public relations game," Motley says, HEAL sent advance teams to meet with reporters in the cities where Senate Majority Leader George Mitchell and other Democrats held hearings in December 1991.

Spending Millions to Promulgate Myths

If they were to tell the truth, the medical and insurance industries would have to admit, "The American health care system may be failing its patients, but we who profit from it are doing very well, and we want to keep it that way. We have a lot of money and use it to hire high-priced lobbyists. We give millions to control legislatures successfully." As the debate escalates, the number of lies will increase and the myths [arguments against reform] will become carefully crafted to emotional 30-second sound bites. But these industries can be beaten if we can explode their myths. And these myths cannot stand in the face of a public highly motivated to assure health care security for ourselves and our loved ones.

MaryAnn O'Sullivan and Nettie Hoge, *Propaganda Review*, Fall 1992, No. 9.

Some observers doubt whether public opinion is forceful or cohesive enough to overcome the money, connections and political savvy of these groups. "There are a lot of interests at risk," says a staff member of the House Energy and Commerce Committee. "Without some clear political constituency that politicians can see and hear and touch and feel it's going to be very hard for them to say they have a clear mandate to move forward on reform.". . .

Significant movement on the issue would require overcoming the insurance companies and small businesses that oppose all but the mildest reform proposals. [They object to a single-payer program like Canada's national health care system, where patients choose their own doctors and receive care in private facilities, but the government acts as the nation's insurance company and imposes strict cost controls. They also dislike attempts to expand the nation's current employment-based health insurance system, where employers would be required to either "pay" the government to enroll their employees in a new public health program or "play" by providing their employees with a minimum package of private health insurance benefits.] A single-payer system would do away with the need for most private health insurance, and insurance executives worry that a pay-or-play system would give employers more incentive to pay into the public program than to provide their employees with private insurance. "We oppose that strenuously, and are working to see that it is not enacted," says David Hebert of the National Association of Life Underwriters.

The Health Insurance Industry's Influence

The Health Insurance Association of America (HIAA), which represents 300 commercial insurance companies that cover some 95 million Americans, "strongly opposes" both pay-or-play and single-payer proposals, says spokesperson Donald White.

To strengthen its hand against federal action, HIAA plans to spend at least $4 million on lobbying, public relations and legal work in 15 "target states." What HIAA does support are "barebones" policies for small businesses, provisions that allow workers to keep their insurance when changing jobs and curbs on the denial of coverage due to preexisting conditions.

The wealth and power of the insurance industry are hard to overstate. "The health insurance industry . . . has tons of money and they love to spend it to get their way on Capitol Hill," says Public Citizen spokesperson Robert Dreyfuss. "In this case they're fighting for their lives.". . .

In addition to the National Association of Life Underwriters, top insurance interests with PACs include the American Family Corp., Travelers, Prudential, Metropolitan Life, Torchmark Corp., CIGNA, HIAA, and Blue Cross and Blue Shield. . . .

Small business also wields big clout. With premiums 25 percent to 40 percent higher than those for larger firms, the cost of health insurance is the "No. 1 problem" of some 500,000 small-business owners, according to the National Federation of Independent Business (NFIB). As a result, many don't provide coverage and don't want to be forced to. They favor tax breaks and lower premiums such as those contained in more limited reform proposals.

The wealthy pharmaceutical companies have been relatively quiet. But should a viable reform plan include coverage and cost controls on prescription drugs, "the drug companies will go crazy" and deploy their lobbyists to defeat it, warns Harvard's Blendon.

That leaves the AMA at the forefront, where doctors will retain their traditional activist role. "You underestimate the AMA's influence at your peril. They have truly awesome power," says AMA member Dr. Quentin Young, a Chicago physician who heads the 4,000-member Physicians for a National Health Program. It supports a Canadian-style, single-payer system. Referring to the influence of the AMA PAC, spokesperson James Stacey says modestly, "We support a large number of congressional candidates. We don't expect that we are buying their minds, their hearts or anything else. Yet we hope that we will have some access to them. The bigger issue is to get physicians involved in the political process.". . .

Misery May Motivate Reform

Grassroots activity is likely to intensify as the health insurance dilemma worsens for individuals and families of all income levels. A Public Citizen study shows that the number of Americans without insurance increased by 1.3 million between 1989 and 1990, with 74 percent of the new uninsured earning more than $25,000 a year. With the economy mired in recession and large-scale layoffs a daily occurrence, workers increasingly worry as much about losing their health benefits as their paychecks.

All of this misery may force Congress to enact some type of reform. "The issue of the uninsured is not enough to move the process," says one congressional aide. "But as the problem becomes worse for the middle class, for working people and people who vote, people will begin to say that this is not acceptable."

"The most important reason costs in the United States surpass those elsewhere is our overuse of medical services."

Overuse of Medical Services Hurts the Health Care System

Edie Rasell

When Americans visit their physicians, they often undergo numerous tests and procedures, many of them unnecessary. This overuse of medical services is a major cause of America's rising health care costs, Edie Rasell argues in the following viewpoint. According to the author, the reasons for this overuse of services range from insurance companies that require physicians to be overly cautious to physicians who intentionally refer patients to labs in which the physician holds a financial interest. Rasell concludes that if the United States is to reform its health care system, it must address the excessive use of medical services. Rasell, a former family physician, is a health economist with the Economic Policy Institute in Washington, D.C., which studies economic policy and promotes education in economics.

As you read, consider the following questions:

1. According to the author, what are the two ways to measure the public's use of medical services, and how do these two ways differ?
2. What reasons does Rasell give for the high intensity of use of medical services in the United States?

From "A Bad Bargain: Why U.S. Health Care Costs So Much and Covers So Few?" by Edie Rasell, *Dollars & Sense*, May 1993. *Dollars & Sense* is a progressive economics magazine published ten times a year. First-year subscriptions cost $16.95 and may be ordered by writing *Dollars & Sense*, One Summer St., Somerville, MA 02143 or calling 617-628-2025.

The U.S. health care system is in crisis. Year by year, fewer people have insurance coverage, while costs skyrocket, draining vital resources from other critical social needs. Family budgets are squeezed and businesses are less competitive internationally. Are we getting our money's worth from this enormous spending? No. Other countries spend much less to provide universal health insurance for their citizens—who also live longer and have fewer infant deaths. And despite years of concern and many "reforms," the U.S. situation is getting worse....

Skyrocketing Costs

Despite the declining rate of insurance coverage, national health care spending is rising rapidly. In 1992 we spent $839 billion for health care, or one-seventh of our Gross Domestic Product (GDP). Adjusted for inflation, spending rose by a whopping 8.5% over 1991, and by 39% since 1987. Since 1988, the share of GDP devoted to health care has risen from 10.8% to 14%.

Health care spending is rising much faster than wages, business receipts, or government revenues. Thus health care is absorbing a growing share of the resources of individuals, firms, and the public sector. Many insurers are requiring people to pay rising portions of their health costs in various forms of cost-sharing, such as deductibles and co-payments. Between 1980 and 1991, the average cost of health insurance for an employee and family rose from $1,806 (in 1991 dollars) to $4,464, while employee out-of-pocket expenses for health care rose from $248 to $1,300.

The United States spends far more on health care than do other industrialized countries, despite having so many people uninsured (see Table 1). In 1990 U.S. per capita spending was nearly 1.5 times the level in Canada, the second highest spending country. Since other countries with lower spending have quite healthy populations and provide coverage for all their people, the United States could spend much less and still have universal, high-quality health care.

Why Costs Are Out of Control

There are two major reasons why the United States has greater spending than other countries—high charges by providers and intensive use of services.

Doctors, hospitals, and other medical providers in the United States charge more for medical care than abroad, and physicians here earn much more than in other countries (see Table 2).

In other industrialized countries, providers and insurers (or a government agency) negotiate fees and charges. The government's goal is to keep medical charges in line with prices in the rest of the economy. In the United States, with the exceptions of Medicare and Medicaid, insurers' usual practice until recently was to pay physicians their "customary and reasonable" rate. This provides little check on price increases. Insurers also reimbursed hospitals based on whatever they charged, not for their actual costs to treat patients.

Part of the reason for high charges by U.S. care providers is huge administrative expenses, totalling 24% of all health spending. In contrast, for Canada's public-insurance system, which covers the entire population, administrative costs are only 11% of the total. Significantly, administrative costs in the U.S. Medicare system are in line with those in other countries. The U.S. Congress' General Accounting Office estimates that in 1991 we would have saved $67 billion if we had had a single insurer, as in Canada.

Table 1: International Health Care Spending, 1990

	Percent of GDP	Per capita
Australia	7.5%	$1,151
Canada	9.0%	$1,795
France	8.9%	$1,379
Germany	8.1%	$1,287
Italy	7.7%	$1,138
Japan	6.5%	$1,145
Sweden	8.7%	$1,421
United Kingdom	6.2%	$932
United States	12.4%	$2,566

Source: *OECD Health Data*, Organization for Economic Cooperation & Development, 1993.

Table 2: Average Physician Income

Canada (1988)	$81,679
Germany (1986)	$86,704
Japan (1989)	$45,324
United Kingdom (1989)	$48,814
United States (1989)	$155,800

Source: *OECD Health Data*, Organization for Economic Cooperation & Development, 1993.

Most of the administrative cost difference stems from the inefficiency of having over 1,500 private health insurance companies selling many different policies in the United States. Each policy may cover different services, restrict enrollees to particular doctors, and impose different levels of cost sharing, different deductibles, and different pre-existing condition exclusions. Administering all of this is an enormous paperwork burden for hospitals, doctors, and insurance companies.

But the most important reason costs in the United States surpass those elsewhere is our overuse of medical services. There are two ways to measure such use. One is *utilization*, which measures the frequency of encounters with the health care system—for example, the average number of doctor visits per person or number of days spent in hospitals. The second is *intensity* of use, which indicates the number and type of services received when someone does visit a doctor or hospital. While high utilization is not a problem in the United States, intensity is the major reason U.S. health care costs surpass those elsewhere.

Compared to other countries, Americans have quite low utilization rates, as shown in Table 3. We average far fewer days in the hospital than do people in any other industrialized country. Visits to the doctor are also less frequent.

Policy-makers and analysts often propose increased cost sharing as a way to discourage utilization and reduce the national health care bill. But since we do not have excessive utilization, this is misguided policy. Forcing further cuts in utilization will only reduce access to necessary care.

Excessive Use of Services

In contrast, the intensity of services used in the United States far surpasses levels in other industrialized countries. Americans do not go to the doctor or enter the hospital very often, but when we do, we receive excessive services compared to people elsewhere.

Intensity of use is high in the United States for several reasons. We have relatively fewer primary-care doctors, and more specialists, than other nations. Specialists tend to order more tests and do more medical procedures. Second, for decades our health care system has rewarded physicians in the United States for "doing" rather than thinking. Payments by insurers for procedures and tests are far higher than for equivalent amounts of time and levels of skill devoted to physical examinations, thinking about solutions to medical problems, talking to patients, or "just" prescribing medicines.

Some doctors who have financial interests in laboratories or radiology facilities order far more tests than those without similar investments. A study of laboratories in Florida, for example, found that those owned by physicians did twice as many tests per patient as did laboratories owned by non-physicians. Another study found that doctors with financial interests in radiology facilities referred patients for x-rays four times more often than did physicians who had not invested in such facilities.

Excess medical equipment and facilities drive up costs in two ways. First, because machines are plentiful, doctors are encouraged to do too many tests. This raises the national health care bill and causes needless pain and suffering. Second, if there are too many machines, then even after doing excessive numbers of tests, the machines are still under-used. For the equipment's owner to recover its purchase price, the charge for each test must be higher than if the machine were fully utilized.

Table 3: Utilization of Services, Annual Average Per Person, 1991

	Hospital Days	Physician Visits
Canada	2.0	6.6
France	2.8	7.1
Germany	3.3	11.5
Japan	4.0	12.9
United Kingdom	2.0	5.3
United States	1.2	5.3

Source: *OECD Health Data*, 1993.

Table 4: Running Up the Tab—Unnecessary Operations

Operation	Appropriate	Equivocal	Inappropriate
coronary angiography	74%	9%	17%
coronary artery bypasses	56%	30%	14%
pacemaker insertion	44%	36%	20%
carotid endarterectomy	35%	32%	32%
endoscopy	72%	11%	17%

(coronary angiography, coronary artery bypasses, and pacemaker insertions are serious procedures done to examine or treat the heart; carotid endarterectomy is surgery on the major arteries in the neck; and endoscopy is a procedure to visualize the interior of the stomach)

Sources: *New England Journal of Medicine* Issue 318; *Journal of the American Medical Association* Issues 258 and 260; *Annals of Internal Medicine* Issue 109.

Another factor that contributes to the high testing rate is the U.S. medical "culture" and the standard of practice taught in medical schools. Many doctors' philosophy is to do everything possible for the patient, to do every test no matter how slim the chance that it will provide useful information. The result is that doctors perform many unnecessary and inappropriate procedures. Several studies reported in medical journals have examined surgical procedures to determine whether they were necessary ("appropriate"), possibly needed ("equivocal"), or unnecessary ("inappropriate"). As Table 4 shows, physicians performed 14% to 32% of selected heart, neck, and stomach procedures for inappropriate reasons, and an additional 9% to 36% were equivocal.

Physicians' practice "style" and local standards of care have a large impact on intensity of use and on medical costs. One study examined services provided by doctors to elder patients in over 300 metropolitan areas. Researchers adjusted for differences between areas in the seriousness of patients' illnesses, and for other factors that influence the need for medical services. Despite these adjustments, differences in the amounts and types of services provided to patients in these cities still resulted in a two-fold difference in spending per patient. Moreover, in those cities where doctors provided more services and costs were higher, patients' health after treatment was no better.

There are several other factors that contribute to our high and rising spending, such as malpractice suits, drug-industry profits, experimental treatments, and the aging of the population. But in contrast to claims made by some medical-care analysts, these factors are only responsible for a small portion of our high and rising expenditures. . . .

But Are We Healthy?

Despite spending more on health care than other industrialized countries, we are not proportionally more healthy. Life expectancy at birth for U.S. females is below the level in 17 other countries, and the rate for men is lower than in 21 other nations. Twenty-two countries, including Italy, Spain, Hong Kong, and Singapore, have a lower infant mortality rate than the United States.

These measures of health depend on more than the health care system. Poverty and the factors that often accompany it, including a poor diet, stress, and dangerous environmental and occupational exposures, all worsen average health in the United States. The lack of prenatal care is a major contributing factor to high infant mortality. The U.S. child immunization rate is lower than in many Third World countries, and has been falling.

Compared to other nations, the United States has an abundance of high-technology medical equipment and facilities, but we impose needless pain and suffering by doing too many tests and procedures. We have too many specialists and too few primary-care physicians. We have helicopter transport to ultrasophisticated trauma units, but little transportation to help rural or inner-city residents reach their family doctors.

The quality of American medical care can be the best in the world, but it also can be very bad. The United States needs a fundamental overhaul of the financing and delivery of health care. We must address the escalating costs, lack of access, and uneven quality of care. And we must remember that a society with high levels of poverty and unemployment can never be a healthy society.

"The erosion of family life . . . drives up the nation's future medical bills."

The Decline of the Traditional Family Has Created a Health Care Crisis

Bryce J. Christensen

Bryce J. Christensen is editor of the *Family in America*, a monthly publication of the Rockford Institute, which supports traditional family values in America. In the following viewpoint, Christensen describes how being married and having children are related to better health. The increase in divorce is reflected in a deterioration of the health of adults and children in America, the author writes. He believes that most of the political proposals for health care reform will further erode family ties, thus worsening the health care crisis.

As you read, consider the following questions:

1. How do family relationships improve one's health and keep medical costs down, according to the author?
2. According to Christensen, in what ways is the health of children affected by the lack of a traditional family structure?
3. Why is America's low birth rate problematic, in the author's opinion?

From "Critically Ill: The Family and Health Care" by Bryce J. Christensen, *The Family in America*, May 1992. Reprinted by permission of the author and the Rockford Institute, Rockford, Illinois.

Health care has pushed itself to the top of the national agenda. In January 1992, Democratic leaders convened a "Town Meeting" on health care in 285 sites around the country. At these town meetings, voters saw a specially prepared video depicting current provisions as wholly inadequate. "We need change, dramatic change," House Speaker Thomas S. Foley (D-WA) says in the tape. Sponsors of the meetings presented three different plans for guaranteeing health care to all Americans. In one option, Medicare would expand to cover all citizens; in a second plan, health care for all Americans would be covered under a new nationalized system, comparable to that found in Canada and many European countries; in a third option (called "play or pay"), the federal government would require all employers either to offer health insurance to their employees or to pay into a national government system for caring for uninsured Americans. Proponents of these systems seek not only to provide all Americans with health care, but also to impose some restraint on runaway health-care costs. Total national health expenditures rose from $74 billion in 1970 to $604 billion in 1989. Real per capita spending on health care has climbed more than five times faster than productivity over the past two decades. The rise in health-care costs paid by government has been even steeper, from $28 billion in 1970 to $190 billion in 1986. The expenses of a single government program—Medicare—have risen from just $7.6 billion in 1970 to $102 billion in 1989. To date, policymakers have achieved only meager success in their efforts to contain costs through price controls, health maintenance organizations, and physician review. National health-care costs are projected to rise to $1.5 trillion by the year 2000 and to a staggering $2 trillion by the year 2030.

Health Linked to Family Life

As pressures grow for a political resolution to the crisis in medical spending, some analysts now believe that the problem cannot be properly understood without considering significant changes in American family life. Although only individual Americans can decide how to order their family lives, a growing body of research reveals that such decisions profoundly affect how much of the nation's wealth must be spent on medical care.

Evidence linking health and family life is not hard to find. Writing in *Social Science and Medicine*, Catherine K. Riessman and Naomi Gerstel observed that "one of the most consistent observations in health research is that married [people] enjoy better health than those of other marital statuses." Riessman and Gerstel noted that "this pattern has been found for every age group (20 years and over), for both men and women, and for both whites and nonwhites.". . .

Demographers at Princeton University have documented the same pattern. In a 1987 study, Ellen S. Kisker and Noreen Goldman analyzed "a range of cultures (Sweden, Japan, England, and Wales, and United States whites)" and found that "in all cases, despite any differences in marriage behavior that may exist, married persons experience lower mortality rates" than single, divorced, and widowed peers. The Princeton team then broadened their survey to 26 developed countries ranging from Austria to New Zealand to Singapore. Across all of those cultures, the results were similar: "It is clear that in developed countries married persons of both sexes experience a marked mortality advantage relative to single individuals." In a 1990 study, Princeton investigators Yuaureng Hu and Noreen Goldman established that in 16 industrialized countries, unmarried men and women suffered from higher death rates than married men and women. The researchers concluded that their findings "strengthen previous speculations about the importance of marriage in maintaining health and the increased stresses associated with both the single and the formerly married states." These findings may be of growing relevance in the years ahead because "for the majority of countries [studied] . . . as well as for both genders, the excess mortality of each unmarried state (relative to married persons) has increased over the past two to three decades."

Singleness Leads to Sickness

Poor health among the unmarried often translates into huge hospital bills, since the unmarried do not have spouses to care for them at home. In a two-year study at the University of Michigan, researchers Lois M. Verbruggs and Donald J. Balaban monitored the health of 165 men and women all aged 55 and over, after their hospitalization for various chronic conditions. The investigators observed that the unmarried men and women suffered from "worse health overall" than the married and spent "far larger fractions of time in the hospital (34.1 percent vs. 16.0 percent)."

And although studies usually find that marriage confers a greater health benefit upon men than upon women, wedlock clearly fosters good health among women, too. In a 1990 study supported by the National Institute of Aging and the National Institute of Mental Health, researchers found that among women ages 40-64, those who were married enjoyed a significant health advantage over those who were unmarried and that those who were mothers were healthier than those without children.

Researchers are still trying to clarify the reasons for the linkage between marriage and good health. . . . Debra Umberson shed more light on the subject in a study published in 1987. She found that mortality rates ran consistently lower for parents

than for adults who are not parents and for the married than for
the unmarried because marriage and parenthood both exert a
"deterrent effect on health-compromising behaviors" such as excessive drinking, drug use, risk-taking, and disorderly living. By
providing a system of "meaning, obligation, [and] constraint,"
family relationships markedly reduce the likelihood of un-
healthy practices.

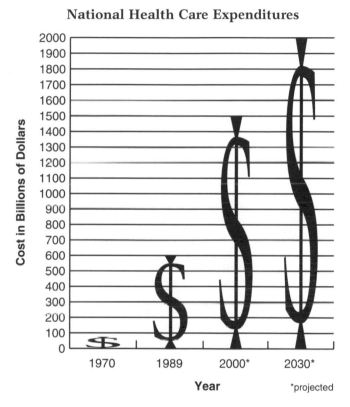

National Health Care Expenditures

Sources: Bureau of the Census, *Statistical Abstract of the United States*, 1991; and *The
Internist*, January 1989.

Evidence of the relationship between divorce and poor health
habits comes from John Clauson of the University of California
at Berkeley. Clauson's research leads him to believe that both
divorce and smoking may be traced to a common personality
profile. According to Clauson, young people with "planful competence" (people who are "thoughtful, self-confident, and responsible") tend to avoid both divorce and smoking, while

47

young people evincing little planful competence tend to become heavy smokers early in life and to divorce in subsequent years.

Yet health habits alone cannot fully account for the health-enhancing effects of marriage. In a study recently completed at Ohio State University, researchers Janice K. Kiecolt-Glaser and colleagues compared the health of separated or divorced men with that of married men who were carefully matched in economic and occupational circumstances. Nor were the two groups distinguishable by "even marginal differences in health-related behaviors." Yet the researchers found that the divorced and separated suffered poorer health and had "poorer cellular immune system control" than their married peers. . . .

Surviving Cancer

In a recent examination of the relationship between marriage and cancer—the nation's second leading cause of death—epidemiologists at the Michigan Cancer Foundation could find no consistent relationship between cancer and marital status (although a statistical relationship between marriage and lower cancer rates could be discerned for a few specific types of cancer such as cancer of the buccal cavity among black and white males and among black females; lung cancer among blacks of both sexes; and cervical and ovarian cancer for females of both races). However, the authors of this study, G. Marie Swanson, Steven H. Belle, and William A. Satariano, did note evidence that "marriage influences survivorship among cancer patients," even if it does not prevent its occurrence. Indeed, in a study conducted in 1987 in New Mexico, researchers found that unmarried victims of cancer are more likely to go untreated for cancer than married victims and even if treated are still less likely to survive than married victims. "The decreases in survival [among cancer victims] associated with being unmarried are not trivial," researchers James S. Goodwin and colleagues noted.

Stressing that "married people live longer and generally are more emotionally and physically healthy than the unmarried," Robert H. Coombs of the UCLA School of Medicine laments that "the therapeutic benefit of marriage remains relatively unrecognized."

Most of the research on the physical health effects of divorce has focused on adults, not children. But parental divorce does appear to put children's health at risk. In *The Broken Heart: The Medical Consequences of Loneliness* (1979), James Lynch of the University of Maryland cited evidence that parental divorce not only causes mental neuroses, but also helps foster "various physical diseases, including cardiac disorders" later in their lives. In a national study in 1985, researchers John Guidubaldi and Helen Cleminshaw found that children of divorced parents suffered significantly worse health than the children of intact marriages. The authors of the study concluded that "marital status is related to health status of all the family members, including both parents and children."

Single Parents and Sick Children

In 1988, researchers Ronald Angel and Jacqueline L. Worobey examined two health surveys conducted by the National Center for Health Statistics, finding that "single mothers report poorer overall physical health for their children." The authors of the study explain their findings by noting that many unmarried mothers live in poverty, so exposing their children to greater health risks, and that a disproportionate number of single mothers are young and therefore more likely to bear an illness-prone premature infant. The Rutgers researchers also uncovered evidence that unmarried mothers are more likely than married mothers to exaggerate the health problems of their children. Indeed, Finnish health authorities at the University of Tampere find that children from broken homes are significantly more likely to require medical attention for psychosomatic symptoms than children from intact families. But most health problems among children in single-parent households are not psychosomatic. In a paper presented in 1990 before the Population Association of America, Deborah Dawson reported that in a national survey, "the overall health vulnerability score was elevated by 20 to 40 percent" among children living with never-married, divorced, and remarried mothers, compared to children living with both biological parents.

Like divorce, illegitimacy appears linked to harmful—often fatal—health problems for children. In a study completed in 1987, researchers Joel C. Kleinman and Samuel S. Kessel at the National Center for Health Statistics found that compared with married mothers, unmarried women run "a substantially higher risk of having infants with very low or moderately low birth weights." Low birth weight defines one of the best predictors of infant mortality. The NCHS researchers believe that marriage exerts no "direct causal influence on the outcome of pregnancy," but argue that a life course that includes marriage is likely to be healthier than one that does not. (Unmarried mothers are, for example, more likely to smoke than married mothers.)

Divorce and illegitimacy also affect the future health of children by increasing the likelihood that they will engage in premarital sex or that they will use tobacco, alcohol, or illegal drugs. In recent studies in the United States and Canada, researchers have shown that, compared to teens from intact homes, adolescents from nonintact families are more likely to engage in premarital sex and to use tobacco, alcohol, and illicit drugs. Such teens appear especially vulnerable to diseases (including AIDS) caused by tobacco, by sexual contact, and by dirty drug needles.

Comparing Mexicans and Puerto Ricans

In another study highlighting the importance of family life on children's health, researchers at Stanford Center for Chicano Research discovered that Mexican-American children are remarkably healthy, significantly more healthy than Puerto-Rican children, even though Mexican Americans are just as impoverished as Puerto Ricans and have much less access to medical care than Puerto Ricans. In trying to explain this "unexpected" pattern, researchers Fernando S. Mendoza and colleagues note a significant difference in family life: "Puerto-Rican families are . . . more likely to be headed by a single parent than Mexican-American families, who have a percentage of two-parent families similar to that of non-Hispanic whites."

"Alternative Lifestyles" and Disease

The deterioration of the family and its influence in American life is arguably the leading cause of disease and premature death. Literally hundreds of studies confirm that marriage and family life enhance health, while divorce, single parenting, cohabitation, homosexuality, and other so-called "alternative lifestyles" increase the likelihood of disease and early death.

Robert W. Lee, *The New American*, June 29, 1992.

American policymakers and concerned citizens can hardly ignore the apparent linkage between family dissolution and poor health at a time of high divorce and illegitimacy rates and of low and falling marriage rates. The American divorce rate has risen more than 40 percent since 1970, by almost 250 percent since 1940. Perhaps 40 percent of marriages formed in the 1980s are headed for divorce. On the other hand, the rate for first marriages among women ages 15-44 has dropped more than 35 percent since 1970; one American in eight now remains unmarried for life. Partly because of a sharp drop in marital fertility, the proportion of the nation's children born out of wedlock has soared. In 1960, only one birth in twenty was illegitimate. In 1985, over one-fourth of all births were out of wedlock.

The health costs associated with this national retreat from family life are not only the burden of individual households, but of the taxpayers. Largely because of the rise in illegitimacy, taxpayers now pay the birth costs for one infant in seven.

Because illegitimate children are born prematurely with alarming frequency, they often require special surgery, mechanical respirators, isolation incubators, and other costly medical care paid for out of general hospital funds and the public purse. In a 1984 study at the National Center for Health Services, analysts Marc L. Berk and Amy K. Taylor found that divorced women were not only less healthy than married women (despite the fact that "the divorced population is somewhat younger than the married"), but that divorced women are more likely than married women to rely on public assistance for health care. Likewise, in their study in 1988 on single motherhood and children's health, researchers Angel and Worobey at Rutgers commented that unmarried mothers and their children "disproportionately constitute a population which is chronically dependent on the state for basic necessities, including health care."

The erosion of family life not only drives up the nation's future medical bills, it also reduces the number of future taxpayers who can pay those bills. Policy analyst Ben Wattenberg identifies the trend toward fewer, later, and less stable marriages as a primary reason for a national fertility rate which has languished below replacement level for more than a decade. Wattenberg indeed believes that the "birth dearth" could cause the Social Security system to fail early in the next century if—as many predict—the Social Security trust fund is combined with the Medicare trust fund.

The Government Provides Care When Families Won't

Family disruption and depressed fertility not only erode the tax base, these developments also create higher public costs for the institutional care of the sick and elderly. In 1977, Lynch reported that Americans were paying "uncounted billions of dollars" to care for divorced and single people who stay in hospitals longer than do married people suffering from the same illnesses. American taxpayers also face rising costs of institutionalizing elderly persons because of childlessness and family dissolution. In RAND Corporation studies published in 1988 and 1990, Peter Morrison warned that trends in American family life may make it difficult to care for the rising number of elderly Americans. He noted that because of high divorce rates, "the care spouses traditionally have provided each other in old age will be far less available" in the decades ahead. The birth dearth will further exacerbate the difficulty of caring for the elderly. "Early next century when baby boomers grow old," Morrison writes, "they will have few adult children to fill the role of caregiver, because they produced so few offspring." And while the working woman's need for paid child care has received a great deal of attention, the plight of the working woman's elderly parents has received less consideration. Pointing out that "by tradition, adult daughters have provided elderly parents with home care," Morrison anticipates a "demographic scenario" in which "elderly Americans long on life expectancy may find themselves short on care where it matters most—at home." Researchers Wayne A. Ray and colleagues from Vanderbilt University anticipated "intergenerational conflict" provoked by the increasing costs of providing nursing-home care for aging Americans without children able or willing to care for them in their homes. In 1989, annual public expenditures for nursing-home care already stood at over $25 billion. Because of the profound effects of marriage and family life upon health-care costs, the public debate over how to meet those costs cannot proceed very far without addressing these issues. That debate is already heating up. Writing in *The New Republic*, Phillip Longman argued that "Medicare is going broke" because of the aging of the population and the declining American birth rate. "Without fundamental changes, Medicare won't be able to meet the needs of today's middle-aged Americans and their children," Longman reasons, warning that under current policies "the trade-off between health care for the young and the old will become increasingly stark and unavoidable." Formerly chief of staff at the White House under President Lyndon Johnson, James R. Jones predicts that unless current trends can be checked, federal spending on health care could consume 20 percent of every American worker's taxable income by the year 2009. Under such a crushing tax burden, younger Americans would find it hard to avoid "a sizable decline in their future standard of living." Jones, therefore, calls for "no less than rethinking our notion of health care entitlement from the bottom up." Fundamental rethinking may account for the rediscovery of family responsibilities by some public-health officials. Richard Morse of Kansas State University sees "some movement, at present, to deny welfare or Medicaid to those individuals whose families cannot prove they are unable to perform that responsibility." Alexa K. Stuifbergen of the University of Texas at Austin likewise believes that "policymakers are increasingly looking to the family as a hedge against the rising cost of health care services.". . .

America's retreat from family life is the consequence of many diverse cultural trends, most of them beyond the direct control of policymakers in a liberal democracy. American government officials are now asked to cope with the rising medical costs created by family dissolution; yet, by collectivizing those costs, these officials help cause further erosion of family ties. It is a dilemma sure to unsettle the nation in the decades ahead.

"There is no health-care crisis."

There Is No Health Care Crisis

Fred Barnes

While many are bemoaning the status of America's health care system, the reality is that Americans have the best health care in the world, Fred Barnes states in the following viewpoint. Barnes acknowledges that health care in America needs some minor improvements, but asserts that no drastic measures are required. Barnes is a senior editor of the *New Republic*, a bi-monthly magazine of political opinion.

As you read, consider the following questions:

1. Why does Barnes contend that uninsured Americans do receive high-quality medical care?
2. Why does the author disagree with the use of life expectancy and infant mortality rates as measures of a nation's health care?
3. What problems does Barnes see in the health care systems of Canada, Japan, Germany, and Great Britain?

Bill and Hillary Clinton have contributed heavily to a national myth. Mrs. Clinton, as boss of the administration task force plotting to overhaul America's health-care system, refers routinely to "the health-care crisis." Her husband uses the same phrase ("Our government will never again be fully solvent until we tackle the health-care crisis," Clinton declared in his 1993 State of the Union address). And he goes one step further. "A lot of Americans don't have health insurance," he told a group of schoolkids during a nationally televised children's town meeting at the White House. "You know that, don't you? A lot of Americans don't have health care."

The press also trumpets the crisis theme. *Parade*, the popular Sunday supplement, emblazoned its cover with this headline: "THE GROWING CRISIS IN HEALTH CARE." The result is that the American people, despite their personal experience, now believe there actually is a health-care crisis. Most opinion polls show roughly three-quarters of Americans are satisfied with the availability and quality of the health care they receive. Yet, in most polls, 60 to 70 percent feel the health-care system is failing and needs significant, if not radical, reform.

Everyone Has Health Care

There is no health-care crisis. It's a myth. If millions of seriously ill Americans were being denied medical care, that *would* be a crisis. But that's not happening. Everyone gets health care in this country—the poor, the uninsured, everyone. No, our health-care system isn't perfect. There isn't enough primary care—regular doctor's visits—for many Americans. Emergency rooms are often swamped. The way hospitals and doctors are financed is sometimes bizarre. Health care may (or may not) be too costly. But it's the best health-care system in the world—not arguably the best, but the best. Its shortcomings can be remedied by tinkering, or at least by less-than-comprehensive changes. An overhaul of the sort Hillary Clinton envisions is not only unnecessary, it's certain to reduce, not expand, the amount of health care Americans receive (price controls always lead to less of the controlled commodity). Then we really will have a health-care crisis.

You don't have to take my word that there's no crisis now and that health care here is the world's best. There's solid evidence. Let's examine four key aspects of the health care debate: access, false measures of quality health care, true measures, and how America's system compares with those of other industrialized democracies (Canada, Germany, Japan, Great Britain).

Will someone please tell Bill Clinton that having no health insurance is not the same as having no health care? The uninsured get health care, only less of it than the insured. Being uninsured means "one is more likely to use emergency-room care and less likely to use office, clinic, or regular inpatient care," said Richard Darman, President Bush's budget director, in congressional testimony in 1991. "This is not to suggest that this is desirable. It is not." But it *is* high-quality health care.

The Best on Earth

All my life I've heard wails against the "crisis" in American health care because of high costs. To this cry I wish to administer a much-needed dose of contrarian skepticism.

Though U.S. health care is not perfect and often excessive, it's still the best on earth. Its high and increasing cost is an expected phenomenon of our modern economy.

Webster Riggs Jr., *American Medical News*, February 10, 1992.

Doctors in emergency rooms are specialists. In fact, they have a professional organization, the American College of Emergency Physicians. Its motto is: "Our specialty is devoted to treating everyone in need, no questions asked." Turning away patients isn't an option. Federal law (section 9121 of the Consolidated Omnibus Budget Reconciliation Act of 1985) requires medical screening of everyone requesting care at a hospital emergency room. If treatment is needed, it must be provided. What this adds up to is "universal access" to health care in America, as one head of a hospital board told me.

It's no secret how much health care the uninsured get. The American Hospital Association estimated in 1991 that hospitals provide $10 billion in uncompensated care annually. Another study found that the 16.6 percent of the non-elderly population who are uninsured—36.3 million people—accounted for 11 percent of the nation's personal health-care expenditures in 1988. They had 37 percent fewer sessions with doctors and 69 percent fewer days in the hospital. There's a reason the uninsured get less health care, beyond the fact most work in low-paying jobs without health insurance. The uninsured tend to be young, thus healthy. According to a new poll by Frederick/Schneiders, 39 percent are 18-29 years of age and another 25 percent are 30-39. By the way, the elderly (65 and up), who require more medical care, are covered. Ninety-nine percent are eligible for Medicare.

Treating AIDS

To make sure we really have universal access, I checked on how victims of the most recent epidemic, AIDS, are treated. These are the folks doctors are supposed to be leery of dealing with.

55

What if a penniless AIDS patient shows up at, say, the
Whitman-Walker Clinic in Washington, D.C.? That patient, even
if indigent, gets treatment. When the time comes (T-cell count
below 500), the patient is started on AZT, which costs about
$5,000 a year. Later, the patient gets expensive, experimental
drugs: DDI, DDC, D-4T. The drugs are paid for mostly by federal funds. There's also doctor care, painkillers, laboratory
work. To prevent infections or complications, the patient is
treated with prophylaxis.

A friend of mine volunteered to help an indigent, bedridden
AIDS patient. He was amazed at the level of care. "It was an
endless supply of extremely sophisticated drugs, an elaborate IV
system [to feed the patient], and eventually a five-day-a-week
home help nurse," my friend said. "Sometimes we had so much
medicine, we had to throw it away. There was never a sense
we'd be left in the lurch." The patient had no insurance. He
lived with a boyfriend, but the boyfriend was not required to pay
for any of the care. The federal and city governments—the taxpayers—footed the bill. The American Medical Association says
"lifetime medical care" for a single AIDS patient costs $102,000.

False Tests

Judging by the two most common measures of health, life expectancy at birth and the infant mortality rate, health care in
the United States is not the best or even among the best. In
1990, life expectancy in America was 72 years for males, 78.8
for women. This put the U.S. behind Canada, France, Germany,
Italy, Japan, and Great Britain, among others. On infant mortality, the U.S. fared still worse, ranking nineteenth in 1989 with a
rate of 9.7. (The infant mortality rate is the number of deaths of
children under one year of age, divided by the number of births
in a given year, multiplied by 1,000.) Finland, Spain, Ireland,
East Germany, and Italy finished higher.

What's wrong with these measures? Just this: they're a reflection of health, not the health-care system. Life expectancy is determined by much more than the quality of a nation's health
care. Social factors affect life expectancy, and this is where the
U.S. runs into trouble. "Exacerbated social problems . . . ad-
versely affect U.S. health outcomes," noted three Department of
Health and Human Services officials in the Fall 1992 issue of
Health Care Financing Review. "The 20,000 annual U.S. homi-
cides result in per capita homicide rates 10 times those of Great
Britain and 4 times those of Canada. There are 100 assaults reported by U.S. emergency rooms for every homicide. About 25
percent of spinal cord injuries result from assaults." And so on.
The incidence of AIDS is even more telling. Through June 1992,
there were 230,179 reported AIDS cases here, two-thirds of

whom have died. Japan, where life expectancy is four years longer for men than in the U.S. and three years longer for women, has had fewer than 300 AIDS cases. Once social factors have played out, the U.S. ranks at the top in life expectancy. At age 80, when most people are highly dependent on the health-care system, Americans have the longest life expectancy (7.1 years for men, 9.0 for women) in the world.

The infant mortality rate (IMR) is also "reflective of health and socioeconomic status and not just health care," wrote four Urban Institute scholars in the summer 1992 issue of *Health Care Financing Review*. And there are measurement problems. Many countries make no effort to save very-low-birth-weight infants. They aren't recorded as "live born" and aren't counted in infant mortality statistics. In contrast, American hospitals make heroic efforts in neonatal intensive care, saving some infants, losing others, and driving up the IMR. "The more resources a country's health-care system places on saving high-risk newborns, the more likely its registration will report a higher IMR," according to the Urban Institute scholars.

A High-Risk Society

Social factors probably have a bigger impact. A poverty rate twice Canada's and Germany's, a rash of drug-exposed babies, a high incidence of unmarried teenage pregnancy— all lead to low-birth-weight infants and affect the IMR. "Infant mortality rates of babies born to unmarried mothers are about two times higher than the rates of babies born to married mothers," the scholars write. The point is not that America's high IMR is excusable, but that it's grown to abnormal levels in large part because of factors unrelated to the quality of health care.

Not only that. The entire medical system bears the brunt of social and behavioral problems that are far worse in the U.S. than in other industrialized democracies. "We have a large number of people who indulge in high-risk behavior," says Leroy L. Schwartz, M.D., of Health Policy International, a non-profit research group in Princeton, New Jersey. Behavioral problems become health problems: AIDS, drug abuse, assaults and violence, sexually transmitted diseases, etc. "The problem is not the health-care system," says Dr. Schwartz. "The problem is the people. Every year the pool of pathology in this country is getting bigger and bigger. We think we can take care of everything by calling it a health problem." But we can't.

Real Tests

While primary and preventive care are important, the best measure of a health-care system is how well it treats the seriously ill. What if you've got an enlarged prostate? Your chances of survival are better if you're treated here. The U.S. death rate from prostate trouble is one-seventh the rate in Sweden, one-fourth that in Great Britain, one-third that in Germany. Sweden, Great Britain, and Germany may have higher incidences of prostate illness, but not high enough to account for the wide disparity in death rates.

Better Care, Higher Costs

Health care is improving more than are many other areas of our economy. This alone could justify its disproportionately increasing cost. Health care providers are now trained longer and better. They are better organized and monitored. Patients are better diagnosed, treated and rehabilitated than in the past. If something improves in quantity or quality its increase in cost is not inflationary and is acceptable. . . .

Americans should understand their chosen expensive health care system as being an expected vital part of our economy that is improving itself as well as their health.

Webster Riggs Jr., *American Medical News*, February 10, 1992.

An ulcer of the stomach or intestine? The death rate per 100,000 persons is 2.7 in the U.S., compared to 2.8 in the Netherlands, 3.1 in Canada, 4.9 in Germany, 7.6 in Sweden, and 8 in Great Britain. A hernia or intestinal obstruction? The American death rate is 1.7. It's 2 in Canada, 2.7 in Germany, 3 in the Netherlands, 3.1 in Great Britain, and 3.2 in Sweden. Can these be attributed solely to varying incidences of ulcers and obstructions? Nope.

Access to Technology

I could go on, and I will. The overall death rate from cancer is slightly higher in America than in Sweden or Germany, but lower than in Canada, the Netherlands, and Great Britain. But for specific cancers, the U.S. has the lowest death rate: stomach cancer, cervical cancer, uterine cancer. Only Sweden has a lower death rate from breast cancer. The U.S. also has the second lowest death rate from heart attack. No matter what the disease—epilepsy, hypertension, stroke, bronchitis—the U.S. compares well. For a country with a heterogeneous population and large pockets of pathology, this is remarkable. Life expectancy for American males at 65 is 14.7 years, only a tad less than Canada (15), Sweden (14.9), and Switzerland (14.9), more homogeneous countries with fewer social problems. (I'm grateful to Dr. Schwartz for all these figures.)

Another measure that's important is the proliferation of new technology. "Major medical technology has had a profound impact on modern medicine and promises even greater impact in the future," wrote Dale A. Rublee, an expert in cross-national health policy comparisons for the AMA's Center for Health Policy Research, in *Health Affairs*. He compared the availability of six technologies—open-heart surgery, cardiac catheterization, organ transplantation, radiation therapy, extracorporeal shock wave lithotripsy, and magnetic resonance imaging—in the U.S., Canada, and Germany in 1987. "Canada and Germany were selected because their overall health-care resources are fairly comparable to the United States," Rublee wrote. The U.S. came out ahead in every category, way ahead in several. In MRI's, the U.S. had 3.69 per one million people, Germany 0.94, Canada 0.46. For open-heart surgery, the U.S. had 3.26, Canada 1.23, Germany 0.74. For radiation therapy, the U.S. had 3.97, Germany 3.13, Canada 0.54. Small wonder that, as Rublee put it, "American physicians, with a universe of modern technology at their fingertips, are the envy of the world's physicians."

Rival Systems

Canadian politicians get special health care privileges, moving to the head of waiting lists or getting treatment at the elite National Defence Medical Centre. But that wasn't sufficient for Robert Bourassa, the premier of Quebec. He came to the National Cancer Institute in Bethesda, Maryland, for diagnosis, then returned to the U.S. for surgery, all at his own expense.

The Canadian health-care system has many nice attributes, but speedy treatment isn't one of them. Ian R. Munro, M.D., a Canadian doctor who emigrated to the U.S., wrote in *Reader's Digest* of a young boy in Canada who needed open-heart surgery to free the blood flow to his lungs. He was put on a waiting list. He got a surgery date only after news reports embarrassed health officials. After waiting two months, he died four hours before surgery. This was an extreme case, but waiting is common in the Canadian system, in which the government pays all costs, including set fees for private doctors. A study by the Fraser Institute in 1992 found that 250,000 people are awaiting medical care at any given time. "It is not uncommon for patients to wait months or even years for treatments such as cataract operations, hip replacements, tonsillectomies, gallbladder surgery, hysterectomies, heart operations, and major oral surgery," according to Edmund F. Haislmaier, the Heritage Foundation's health-care expert. Canada has other problems: health costs are rising faster than in the U.S., hospital beds and surgical rooms are dwindling, and doctors are fleeing (8,263 were practicing in the U.S. in 1990).

The Japanese model isn't any better. When Louis Sullivan, M.D., President Bush's secretary of health and human services, visited Japan, he was surprised to find medical care matched that of the U.S.—the U.S. of the 1950s. Japan has universal access and emphasizes primary care at clinics, financed mostly through quasi-public insurance companies. The problem is price controls. "Providers seek to maximize their revenue by seeing more patients," wrote Naoki Ikegami, professor of health at Keio University in Tokyo. "This dilutes the services provided."

Patients receive assembly-line treatment. "In outpatient care, a clinic physician sees an average of 49 patients per day [and] 13 percent see more than 100," Ikegami said. For the elderly, a survey found, the average number of doctor's visits for a six-month period was 17.3 (3.6 here) and the length of visits was 12 minutes (30 in the U.S.). Like Canada's queues, this is an extraordinarily inefficient way to dispense care. Patients return repeatedly to get the same care that in the U.S. is given in a single visit.

Bribes to Doctors

Japanese doctors also prescribe and sell drugs. Not surprisingly, they sell plenty. Thirty percent of the country's health expenditures are for drugs (7 percent in the U.S.). In Japan, wrote Ikegami, "no real incentives exist to maintain quality." The one exception is specialists at Japan's teaching hospitals. To avoid queues, patients pay bribes of $1,000 to $3,000 to be admitted to a private room and treated by a senior specialist.

Germany also has strict fees for doctors, with predictable results. Annual doctor's visits per capita are 11.5 (5.3 here), a figure exceeded only by Japan (12.9). In other words, price controls are as inefficient in Germany as in Japan. Hospitals face perverse incentives, too. The government pays a fixed rate per day, regardless of the patient's illness or length of stay. So hospitals pad their billings by keeping patients for unnecessarily long recuperations, which compensates for the losses they incur taking care of critically ill patients.

Then there's Great Britain, home of the National Health Service. Officials take great pride in having reduced the number of patients waiting more than two years for medical attention. In 1986, the number was 90,000; in 1991, 50,000. In April 1992, it was down to 1,600. Sounds great, but there's a catch. The number of patients waiting six months or less grew by 10 percent. The overall drop in waiting lists was only 3 percent. And this was achieved, a survey by the National Association of Health Authorities and Trusts found, chiefly because of a 13 percent hike in NHS spending in 1991, not increased efficiency. The good news in Great Britain is that private insurance is allowed and 6.6 million Brits have it. Insurance firms encourage beneficiaries to have an operation or other treatment in a private hospital. Sure, the company pays, but it knows that once a patient has experienced care in a private hospital, he'll never go back to the socialized medicine of NHS. And he'll keep buying health insurance. Private hospitals, anxious to fill empty beds, have their own come-on. At Christmas, they offer discount prices for operations.

Europe Looks to the United States

In truth, the U.S. has little but painful lessons to learn from the health-care experience of other countries. There's practically nothing to emulate. On the contrary, foreign health officials, Germans especially, now look at the incentives in the American medical system as a way to remedy problems in their health-care systems. Hillary Clinton and health policy wonks should stop apologizing for our system.

They won't. The existence of a few health-care problems, chiefly the lack of proper primary care for several million Americans, allows them to declare a crisis and go on wartime footing. Liberals love this. . . . The program that emerges is sure to dwarf the problem. If enacted, it will make the problem worse. This is a common phenomenon in Washington. Some people never learn.

In 1991, an American official addressed Russian health experts in Moscow. He bemoaned that many Americans get care at emergency rooms and occasionally wait six or eight hours. To the American's shock, the Russians erupted in laughter. In Russia, with twice as many doctors per capita as the U.S., a wait of six to eight hours represented unusually fast service.

61

Periodical Bibliography

The following articles have been selected to supplement the diverse views presented in this chapter.

Marcia Angell "How Much Will Health Care Reform Cost?" *The New England Journal of Medicine*, June 17, 1993. Available from the Massachusetts Medical Society, 1440 Main St., Waltham, MA 02254.

Dan E. Beauchamp "Universal Health Care, American Style: A Single Fund Approach to Health Care Reform," *Kennedy Institute of Ethics Journal*, Vol. 2, No. 2, 1992. Available from Johns Hopkins University Press, 701 W. 40th St., Suite 275, Baltimore, MD 21211.

Judith Bell "Why Competition Won't Cure America's Health-Care Ills," *Business & Society Review*, Winter 1993.

Daniel Callahan "Our Fear of Dying," *Newsweek*, October 4, 1993.

Barbara Ehrenreich "We Have Seen the Enemy: It Isn't Us," *Health/PAC Bulletin*, Summer 1993. Available from 853 Broadway, Suite 1607, New York, NY 10003.

Edmund Faltermayer "Let's *Really* Cure the Health System," *Fortune*, March 23, 1992.

William H. Foege "Preventive Medicine and Public Health," *Journal of the American Medical Association*, July 15, 1992. Available from Subscriber Services Center, American Medical Association, 515 N. State St., Chicago, IL 60610.

Edmund F. Haislmaier "Why Global Budgets and Price Controls Will Not Curb Health Costs," *The Heritage Foundation Backgrounder*, March 8, 1993. Available from 214 Massachusetts Ave. NE, Washington, DC 20002-4999.

James A. Rice "What's Right and Wrong with U.S. Health Care," *The World & I*, June 1992.

David J. Rothman "A Century of Failure: Health Care Reform in America," *Journal of Health Politics, Policy and Law*, Vol. 18, No. 2, Summer 1993. Available from Duke University Press, 6697 College Station, Durham, NC 27708.

2 CHAPTER

Have Physicians Hurt America's Health Care System?

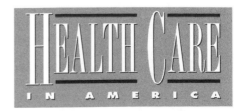

Chapter Preface

The relationship between patients and their physicians has been eroding in the last few decades, in the opinion of many Americans. "Trust between doctor and patient has broken down on both sides. Increasingly cold and transient encounters characterize what was once called healing," laments physician and professor Melvin Konner. Many Americans agree with Konner, according to a 1991 Gallup Poll: Almost 70 percent of respondents felt that Americans are losing faith in their physicians.

One issue that angers many patients is physicians' high fees: In a March 1993 *Newsweek* poll, 83 percent of respondents said they believed physicians charge too much. In 1991, the median net income for physicians was $140,090; the average median income for all occupations was $22,360. "I don't think the American public has a great deal of sympathy for physician incomes that are six times what the average worker receives, and rising at rates far in excess of what other workers are receiving," concludes consumer advocate Ron Pollack. In addition, some critics accuse physicians of performing unnecessary surgery and ordering useless tests and procedures simply to increase their earnings or to protect themselves from malpractice lawsuits. These suspicions have decreased the respect Americans have long held for physicians and have caused a breach in the patient-physician relationship.

Physicians in turn feel unappreciated and unfairly attacked. They defend their salaries, arguing that their work requires extensive education—four years of college, four years of medical school, a year as an intern, and three to ten years as a resident, depending on the specialty. "Physicians have an enormous investment in their education. As a group, they frequently have responsibility for the life or death of patients," attests physician Harry Schwartz. And Melvin Konner believes Americans should support and thank their physicians: "Doctors are not the enemy. They are the officer corps of our own health care army. . . . Most are making low to reasonable incomes doing the hardest job in the world—and the one that requires the most training. We have got to stop attacking them." Konner and others assert that, if doctors do practice defensive medicine—that is, order excessive tests and procedures—it is because they fear unfair lawsuits from patients. Doctors, physician Naomi Bluestone writes, work hard—an average of sixty hours a week—and consequently "deserve to be nurtured, not taken for granted and abused. Their work . . . is stressful, difficult, and exhausting."

The authors in the following chapter attempt to identify the causes of the rift between physicians who feel unappreciated and patients who feel alienated and seek ways to heal it.

"We cannot expect to solve our health-care problems unless we can count on the basic altruism of the [medical] profession."

Physicians Have Contributed to a Health Care Crisis

Arnold S. Relman

Arnold S. Relman is a professor of medicine and social medicine at Harvard Medical School in Cambridge, Massachusetts, and editor-in-chief emeritus of the *New England Journal of Medicine*. In the following viewpoint, Relman argues that physicians have changed from being caring professionals concerned about patients' needs to entrepreneurs concerned only about profit. The author concludes that America's health crisis will end only when physicians rediscover the profession's goal of serving the public good.

As you read, consider the following questions:

1. Why must physicians compete for patients, according to Relman?
2. What are the consequences of increased specialization and technological sophistication in medicine, according to the author?
3. What does Relman believe will happen if America's health care system continues to be commercialized?

From "What Market Values Are Doing to Medicine" by Arnold S. Relman. Reprinted from *National Forum: The Phi Kappa Phi Journal*, vol. 73, no. 3, Summer 1993, © 1993 by Arnold S. Relman, by permission of the publishers.

Until recently . . . most people considered medical care to be a social good, not a commodity, and physicians usually acted as if they agreed. Physicians were not impervious to economic pressures, but the pressures were relatively weak and the tradition of professionalism was relatively strong.

This situation is now rapidly changing. In the past two decades or so health care has become commercialized as never before, and professionalism in medicine seems to be giving way to entrepreneurialism. The health-care system is now widely regarded as an industry, and medical practice as a competitive business. Let me try briefly to explain the origins and describe the scope of this transformation.

Competition for Patients

First, the past few decades have witnessed a rapid expansion of medical facilities and personnel, leading to an unprecedented degree of competition for paying patients. Our once too few and overcrowded hospitals are now too numerous and on average less than 70 percent occupied. Physicians, formerly in short supply and very busy, now abound everywhere (except in city slums and isolated rural areas), and many are not as busy as they would like to be. Professionalism among self-employed private practitioners thrives when there is more than enough to do. When there isn't, competition for patients and worry about income tend to undermine professional values and influence professional judgment. Many of today's young physicians have to worry not only about getting themselves established in practice but also about paying off the considerable debt they have accumulated in medical school. High tuition levels make new graduates feel that they have paid a great deal for an education that must now begin to pay them back—handsomely. This undoubtedly influences the choice of specialty many graduates make and conditions their attitudes toward the economics of medical practice.

Along with the expansion of health care has come a great increase in specialization and technological sophistication, which has raised the price of services and made the economic rewards of medicine far greater than before. With insurance available to pay the bills, physicians have powerful economic incentives to recruit patients and provide expensive services. In an earlier and less technologically sophisticated era, most physicians were generalists rather than specialists. They had mainly their time and counsel to offer, commodities that commanded only modest prices. Now a multitude of tests and procedures provide lucrative opportunities for extra income. This inevitably encourages an entrepreneurial approach to medical practice and an overuse of services. . . .

Physicians . . . struggle to maintain their income in an increasingly competitive economic climate. Like hospitals, practicing physicians have begun to use advertising, marketing, and public-relations techniques to attract more patients. Until recently, most medical professional societies considered self-promotion of this kind to be unethical, but attitudes have changed, and now competition among physicians is viewed as a necessary, even beneficial, feature of the new medical marketplace.

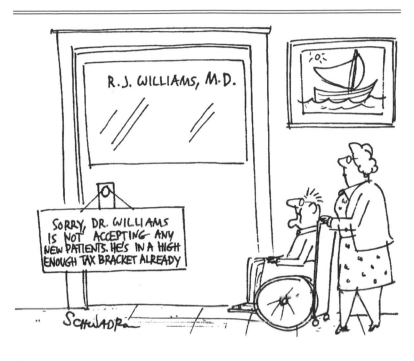

© Harley Schwadron. Reprinted with permission.

Many financially attractive opportunities now exist for physicians to invest in health-care facilities to which they can then refer their patients, and a growing number of doctors have become limited partners in such enterprises—for example, for-profit diagnostic laboratories and magnetic resonance imaging (MRI) centers, to which they refer their patients but over which they can exercise no professional supervision. Surgeons invest in ambulatory surgery facilities that are owned and managed by businesses or hospitals and in which they perform surgery on their patients. Thus they both are paid for their professional services and share in the profits resulting from the referral of their patients to a particular facility. A study in Florida revealed that approximately 40 percent of all physicians practicing in that state had financial interests in facilities to which they referred patients. The AMA [American Medical Association], however, estimates that nationwide the figure is about 10 percent.

In other kinds of entrepreneurial arrangements, office-based practitioners make deals with wholesalers of prescription drugs and sell those drugs to their patients at a profit or buy prostheses from manufacturers at reduced rates and sell them at a profit—in addition to the fees they receive for implanting the prostheses. In entering into these and similar business arrangements, physicians are trading on their patients' trust. This is a clear violation of the traditional ethical rule against earning professional income by referring patients to others or by investing in the goods and services recommended to patients. Such arguments create conflicts of interest that go far beyond the economic conflict of interest of the fee-for-service system, and they blur the distinction between business and the medical profession. . . .

Why Should the Public Care?

The quality and effectiveness of our medical care depend critically on the values and the behavior of its providers. If health care is not a business, then we should encourage our physicians to stand by their traditional fiduciary obligations, and we should enable, if not require, our voluntary hospitals to honor their commitments to the community.

If most of our physicians become entrepreneurs and most of our hospitals and health-care facilities become businesses, paying patients will get more care than they need and poor patients will get less. In a commercialized system, the cost of health care will continue to escalate, and yet we will not be assured of getting the kind of care we really need. In such a system we will no longer be able to trust our physicians, because the bond of fiduciary responsibility will have been broken. To control costs, government will be driven to adopt increasingly stringent regulations. Ultimately health care will have to be regulated like a public utility, and much greater constraints will be placed on physicians and hospitals than are now in place or even contemplated.

Our health-care system is inequitable, inefficient, and too expensive. It badly needs reform. The task will be arduous, and the solution is far from clear; but I believe that the first step must be to gain a firm consensus on what we value in health care and what kind of a medical profession we want. The medical profession has held a privileged position in American society, based on the expectation that it will serve society's needs first of all. How can it hope to continue in that position if it loses the trust of the public? We cannot expect to solve our health-care problems unless we can count on the basic altruism of the profession and its sense of responsibility to patients and the welfare of the general public. American society and the medical profession need to reaffirm their *de facto* contract because they will have to depend on each other as the United States painfully gropes its way toward a better system of health care.

Physicians have the power to make health-care reform possible. They know the system better than anyone, and if they want, they can use its resources more prudently than they do now without any loss of medical effectiveness. It is primarily their decisions that determine what medical services will be provided in each case, and therefore what the aggregate expenditure for health care will be. If physicians remain free of conflicting economic ties, and if they act in a truly professional manner, medical facilities will probably be used more appropriately, regardless of their ownership or organization. In any case, no proposed reforms in the health-care system can ultimately be successful without a properly motivated medical profession. But if physicians continue to allow themselves to be drawn along the path of private entrepreneurship, they will increasingly be seen as self-interested businessmen and will lose many of the privileges they now enjoy as fiduciaries and trusted professionals. They will also lose the opportunity to play a constructive role in shaping the major reforms that are surely coming.

"Physicians are personally getting the blame for the confusing state of insurance affairs."

Physicians Are Blamed Unfairly for the Crisis

Tim Norbeck

The insurance industry, not physicians, is to blame for America's health care crisis, Tim Norbeck asserts in the following viewpoint. Norbeck contends that most Americans are pleased with the quality of care they receive from their personal physicians, but are unhappy with the system that pays for the care. The author believes that radical changes in the insurance industry are necessary to improve health care in America. Norbeck is executive director of the Connecticut State Medical Society.

As you read, consider the following questions:

1. What role do the news media play in Americans' perceptions about health care, in Norbeck's opinion?
2. How are other nations' health care systems better than America's, according to the author?
3. What does Norbeck believe physicians must do to defend their reputations?

"What Is the *Real* Cause of U.S. Complaints About Health Care?" by Tim Norbeck, *American Medical News*, April 20, 1992. Reprinted with the author's permission.

All of us in the federation of medicine are frustrated by the polls indicating that, on one hand, a substantial majority of the American public appears very satisfied with their own physician and the care received, but on the other hand, they are distrustful of physicians as a group. For example, the AMA's public opinion poll of 1991 indicates that the public's favorable opinion of an individual's own personal doctor is rising. At the same time, there was some slippage of an already somewhat low opinion of doctors in general. This difference between the public's opinion of personal physicians and doctors in general is called the "image gap," and it's widening.

Of course, Congress has the same problem but to a worse degree. For example, a *New York Times*/CBS News Poll indicates that 69% of those queried said they disapproved of the way Congress was handling its job—but in the same poll, 51% said they approved of their own representative. This gap has been explained as an anti-institution bias that the American people have.

But can that reason really explain the extraordinary gap of 59 points in the AMA poll? Here, some 69% agreed with the statement that "people are beginning to lose faith in doctors," while only 10% said that about their own doctor. A strong reason for this larger gap must be the pervasive influence of the news media.

As *New York Times* reporter Steven Holmes has suggested, with newspaper, radio and television constantly focusing people's attention on national woes, the public begins to believe that it really is a jungle out there. Yet what is seen on the nightly news or on the front page of the newspaper often does not square with one's own experience.

Doctor-Bashing by the Media

Frank Newport, editor-in-chief of the Gallup Poll, explains it this way: "When asked for a quick response over the telephone, people have to immediately find a frame of reference. They first go from experiential data—their own lives and their community," he says. "But when assessing what's happening around the nation and the world, they can't use experiential data. They must use other sources of information, i.e., what they've seen in the media." And we know how both media and government engage in unceasing doctor-bashing.

Part of the image problem may be due to the fact that most of the newspapers today have been swallowed up by media conglomerates. In 1940, all of the newspapers in the United States were locally owned and independent. Today only 398 remain so, and the other 1,233 are "group" newspapers and no longer locally owned. I can't help thinking that medicine's image has worsened over this period partly because the "national" view

71

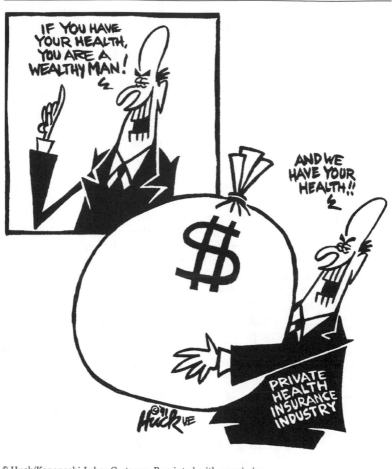

© Huck/Konopacki Labor Cartoons. Reprinted with permission.

has taken over any independent thoughts.

As for television, the number of nightly news stories about health on the three major networks grew from 354 in 1989 to 629 in 1990. It would not surprise me if the growth in 1991 were comparable. The greater the "national" coverage, the worse physicians seem to fare in the reporting. We have all heard the expression "No news is good news." Those in the media seem to have twisted that around to read "Good news is no news." Reporting only the bad news is disinformation rather than information.

As critics so fondly remind us, surveys indicate that the American public is not happy with our health care system. In a recent 10-country survey that some of them happily refer to, only Italy had the same degree of dissatisfaction as expressed by the American public. But this dissatisfaction, if you will, over our system is not really related to the delivery part. Nor is it related to costs inasmuch as surveys indicate that the public wants more money spent on health care, not less. All the polls indicate that a substantial majority of the American public are very satisfied with their care and their physicians.

The Insurance System Is to Blame

If neither the cost of American health care nor its quality are the source of dissatisfaction with our health care system, then that dissatisfaction must be rooted in the insurance system by which the care is financed. In 38 different surveys taken betwen 1988 and 1992, when asked, "Are you satisfied with the medical care that you receive?" most answered yes. On the question "Do you view this care at least as excellent or good?" 81% said "yes" and only 3% said they viewed it as "poor." But when asked, "What do you think of the American health care system?" suddenly the high ratings drop to 35%.

When people talk of rebuilding or the need for fundamental reform of our system, Princeton health economist Uwe Reinhardt, PhD, emphasizes that they are talking about our health insurance system.

As he points out, countries whose citizens give their health care system a high rating provide those citizens with secure health insurance coverage that is portable between jobs and localities and whose premium is divorced from the individual's health status. Their citizens don't worry about a job-lock, that fear of changing jobs because of a previous medical history. Their cancer patients don't worry about a waiting period before they can secure coverage. Their insurance systems are administratively simple. In comparison, our insurance policies are confusing, not portable and are priced to reflect the health status of the individual.

The rest of the world seems to feel that it is repugnant to charge higher premiums for someone just because that someone is unfortunate enough to have a special illness. The rest of the world wouldn't deny someone health insurance protection just because that someone is afflicted with poor health.

The Difference Between the System and the Care

Physicians are being blamed for all these happenings and shortcomings—mainly because the American public and legislators do not understand the issues involved. Physicians are personally getting the blame for the confusing state of insurance affairs. It will be of paramount importance for us to make clear to

73

the public and our legislators the contrast between people's dissatisfaction over our health care insurance system and the satisfaction with the care itself. If we fail to make that distinction, whatever health care reform is enacted will include further harmful intrusions into the practice of medicine.

Physicians throughout the country support the concept of health insurance for all Americans but not through "planned scarcity" or rationing schedules that replace physicians' medical judgment. AMA's "Health Access America" plan has led the charge for more coverage, but not less care. . . .

It will be important for physicians to reach out to all social and service clubs in America and seize every other opportunity to set the record straight and to represent medicine's position on health care insurance reform. There is a story to be told but we cannot depend on others to tell it. As former House Speaker Tip O'Neill said at an AMPAC forum at the AMA Annual Meeting, "Physicians may have many problems, but remember that everyone still respects you more than anyone else. You have instant credibility in your communities."

It is imperative that we utilize that credibility. As Henry V uttered while planning a victory against a foe that outnumbered him five to one: "All things are ready, if our minds be so."

"Physician fees are rising at a 15% annual rate, even though normal inflation is less than six percent."

Physicians Are Too Greedy

Charles B. Inlander

In the following viewpoint, Charles B. Inlander compares American physicians to vultures preying on consumers. He believes physicians are greedy and uncaring, and concerned only with increasing their income and protecting their reputations. Inlander is president of the People's Medical Society, a consumer advocacy organization based in Allentown, Pennsylvania.

As you read, consider the following questions:

1. How did physicians manage to thrive during the recession of the early 1980s, in the author's opinion?
2. How are women in particular victims of physicians, according to Inlander?
3. How have hospitals colluded with physicians and thereby harmed patients, in Inlander's opinion?

"The Hovering Vultures: How Greedy Physicians Prey Upon Patients" by Charles B. Inlander. Reprinted, with permission, from *USA Today* magazine, July 1993. Copyright 1993 by the Society for the Advancement of Education.

In the desert, when a distressed animal is on the verge of death, vultures gather above. This hovering horde of bone pickers sense, with great precision, the near-terminal condition of the creature. Patiently, with uncanny determination, the birds plot their moves. Then, at the very minute they witness the last gasp of their would-be feast, they strike. In short order, they have engorged their victim, ravenously consuming everything edible that hangs from the carcass. Finally, they depart, but behind they have left a warning, maybe meant as a boast. Scattered across the desert floor are the bones of their prey. Left to decay in the hot sun, they remain as a sign to the rest of us that another creature is just waiting to take advantage of our suffering.

Not all vultures operate in the desert, nor are they all winged creatures of the *Cathartidae* family, identified by their dark plumage and naked head and neck. Some can be identified by their white coats, luxurious automobiles, and average after-tax income of $120,000. Many have the initials M.D. or D.O. after their name. They often are spotted at meetings of local or state medical societies. Many migrate to warm-weather resorts in the winter or to Chicago in the summer—the nesting sites of the American Medical Association's conventions.

Even if you do not spot these vultures visually, you may hear them. They often perch on radio talk shows or leave their verbal droppings in the local newspaper. While their chirping tune can vary, it generally is recognized by complaints about Medicare reimbursement, patients' lawsuits, failure of consumers to understand how tough it is for birds of their feather, and the lack of respect most mortals have for such an important species. Indeed, it is this species—the *Vulture Medicus*—who today pose a very serious threat to most American consumers.

Doctor-Vultures Thrived in Recession

While economists are in dispute about whether we remain in a recession, the *Vulture Medicus* continues to stalk its prey, having spotted indicators on the nightly news. The stock market is highly volatile. Oil prices are creeping back up. Housing starts remain at long-time lows. Interest rates are down, meaning invested income earns less. Unemployment still is rising. Companies are delaying expansion. Truck and auto manufacturers are shutting down plants. Steel manufacturers are hurting and making joint deals with foreign competitors. To the *Vulture Medicus*, these signs are a call to hover. While the rest of society gives in or gives up, the *Vulture Medicus* is planning its move. Americans should take heed. The bones from its previous attack still are out there. They have been bleaching in the sun since the last recession and cannot be ignored.

The *Vulture Medicus* remembers the early 1980s, recalling how

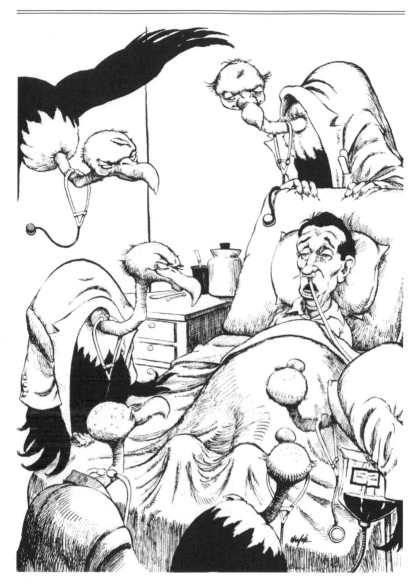

From *USA Today*, July 1993. Reprinted with permission.

companies fired hundreds of thousands of medically insured workers. Consumers came to its office less likely to accept the creature's suggestion to have some elective surgery done. This creature saw costs rise, but the number of patients remain static. So, it raised prices, making sure to keep its increases at least twice that of normal inflation. Why should *Vulture Medicus* have to alter its lifestyle? *Vulture Medicus* is smarter than steel workers, craftier than car salesmen, and more deserving of the good life than teachers or municipal workers. In the early 1980s, when many of these people put the word "former" before their occupational description, *Vulture Medicus* flourished. Its income rose. Hospitals were giving it bonuses to bring in more patients. The creature started its own laboratory, dispensed medication in its own office, maybe even bought a free-standing emergency center.

Vulture Medicae

Life was so good that more *Vulture Medicae* were bred. In fact, the number hatched since 1980, compared to the growth of the general population, has caused most major metropolitan areas to be overrun by the species. Some experts argue that their numbers constitute as big a public health hazard as their pigeon relatives. Only a glut of *Vulture Medicae* can account for the creation of such medical specialties as sports gynecology or sports medicine.

The signs of another *Vulture Medicus* attack are emerging. They are complaining to the government about being overregulated. They carp about patients who cannot afford to pay. They come on the radio or write to "Letters to the Editor" columns whining about the enormous increases in their cost of doing business. They have the unmitigated gall to acknowledge that they overtest and perform unnecessary surgery, all in the name of self-defense.

Women seem to be particularly prime pickings. Ornithologists may attribute this to the three-to-one ratio of male *Vulture Medicae* to the female variety. Whatever the reason, the facts are clear: The female human is the most obvious victim.

For instance, 25% of all babies born in America are delivered by Cesarian section. In 1970, only 5% of births were surgically assisted. England, with an 11.5% C-section rate, considers that number to be a national disgrace, brimming on scandal. The defensive medicine argument doesn't hold up in the C-section fiasco. In places where hospitals have made concerted efforts to monitor unnecessary C-sections, some rates have dropped by as much as 50%. Some insurers—the principal feed providers to the species—have started paying the subspecies *Vulture Obstetricus* the same amount whether the delivery was a natural one or a Cesarian. Figures on the effect of such financing changes show a drop in C-sections.

The examples of women as choice game are many. Experts suggest that more than half the hysterectomies performed are unnecessary. The number of tranquilizers prescribed to females is three times those doled out to males. . . .

The human male is not immune as prey. Thirty percent of all coronary bypass operations, most of which are undergone by men, are considered unnecessary. Certain prostate procedures now are coming under suspicion as being performed inappropriately in many situations.

Even young members of the human species are caught in this apparent campaign of greed. Tonsils are being removed unnecessarily. Circumcisions are being performed when not medically or hygienically essential. Tubes are being placed in far more children's ears than clinically called for.

It is clear that, like their winged brothers, *Vulture Medicae* shows no mercy for their victims. Physician fees are rising at a 15% annual rate, even though normal inflation is less than 6%. . . .

Vulture Medicae are crafty old birds. They have worked hard over the years to develop a beautiful coat of feathers that covers an often ruthless personality. . . . Yet, beneath that surface of fine plumage often lurks a self-centered, hawk-like personality. Too many of the species are inconsiderate and uncaring. Some keep their prey stewing for hours on end, trapped in a chamber with other sick creatures. Their assistants, canaries in white, try to calm the soon-to-be-victim with phrases like "The Vulture has an emergency! While we're waiting, let's fill out some insurance forms," or "The Vulture is running behind. Just be patient." In reality, many merely are on the phone with another shrewd bird, plotting a business investment.

Studies of the *Vulture Medicus* report a changing bird. The education received from its elders is more technical than human. The *Vulture Medicus* has become so impersonal that many hospitals are using ink markers on patients before they are sent down to the surgical suite to avoid the *Vulture Medicus* performing the wrong procedure. All this transpires because the *Vulture Medicus* too often views its game as a condition, rather than a person. It is not unusual for a hospitalized patient to hear himself or herself referred to as the "gallbladder in room 405."

Collusion with Hospitals

Hospitals are where the species loves to hang out since they provide a wealth of devices and equipment for its free use. It's a game that hospitals play in order to attract the best of the breed. Often, however, best of the breed doesn't equate to the best medical results. It merely may mean providing the largest amount to the bottom line. Indeed, the *Vulture Medicus* who admits the most patients or does the most high-volume, expensive procedures is treated like royalty. An entire hospital wing (no pun intended) may be dedicated to this pillar of the community.

Talon to talon, hospitals and *Vulture Medicus* work together. They often collude to keep important information out of the hands of the general public. Very few people are told what a hospital infection rate is. Hardly a soul knows how many medication errors a hospital makes in a day. When a member of the inner gaggle decides to squawk about an incompetent, fellow old coot, the species circles and goes right for the eyes, ears, nose, and throat of the bird with the loud caw. What results is a broken bird, with no referrals, less privileges, and few friends. Other birds see this and decide to keep closed-beaked forever.

Curbing Physicians' Power

There is no question that *Vulture Medicus* is a powerful creature, but there are signs that its strength is weakening. Since the middle 1960s, the species has lost many big battles. It started with Medicare, which the entire *Medicus* family opposed. They screeched that Medicare would be the demise of quality medical care. It was the first step to a "socialized" medical system and would hurt, rather than help, the public, they maintained.

As it turned out, Medicare proved a godsend to the *Vulture Medicus*. The program guaranteed that the often sickest members of society now would be able to pay for medical care. Not only did it mean that elderly Americans had access to medical services, it also signified that *Vulture Medicus* could give its charity to a place that could put its name on a plaque, rather than have to provide medical care to some poor elderly soul.

Of course, *Vulture Medicus* opposed health maintenance organizations. Such programs took the "peck-them-while-they're-down" fun out of medicine. HMOs meant *Vulture Medicus* would be paid a salary or a set fee that didn't reward unnecessary tests and procedures. That was a whole new tree to get used to, but *Vulture Medicus* has had to do so.

Today, *Vulture Medicus* continues trying to exert its power. The American Medical Association has offered its plan to assure full access to health care to all Americans. With 37,000,000 uninsured Americans, the *Vulture Medicus* has a lot at stake. Just think what life could be like if 37,000,000 more potential people were available for the picking. It makes even the nicest of birds sharpen its beak.

The victim of the vulture in the desert usually is helpless when the hovering begins. Nothing short of a miracle can save the wretched prey from the talons and beak of its predator. However, we do not have to be the victim of *Vulture Medicae*. We are not down nor are we helpless. We must ignore their cackling and take charge ourselves. *Vulture Medicus* is a family of predators that can be tamed in the marketplace, halls of state and Federal legislative bodies, and offices of the tax-paid public servants who oversee the rules and regulations that govern medicine.

All species of vulture hover only if there is a victim soon to be had. Without victims, the predator either must change its ways or die off. Our job is not to be a victim.

"Many Americans wrongly believe that profiteering doctors are the major cause of high medical costs. "

Physicians Are Not Greedy

Mike Royko

Mike Royko is a nationally syndicated columnist who writes for the *Chicago Tribune* daily newspaper. In the following viewpoint, Royko defends physicians' high salaries. He asserts that physicians are not greedy, and that those who criticize physicians do not understand how much education, expense, and hard work goes into becoming a physician and into practicing medicine. Smoking, excessive eating and drinking, drug use, and a lack of exercise are the real reasons for America's high health care costs, Royko adds. He concludes that Americans should change their lifestyles if they really want health care costs to go down.

As you read, consider the following questions:

1. What emotions motivate Americans who believe physicians are overpaid, in Royko's opinion?
2. What qualifications to become a physician does Royko list?
3. What course of action does the author suggest for those who think physicians are overpaid?

"Doctors' Pay Poll Is 'Stupid,' Reflects Sick Society," *American Medical News*, May 3, 1993. This article originally appeared in the April 1, 1993, *Chicago Tribune* and is reprinted by permission: Tribune Media Services.

On a stupidity scale, a recent poll about doctors' earnings is right up there. It almost scored a perfect brain-dead 10.

It was commissioned by some whiny consumers group called Families USA. The poll tells us that the majority of Americans believe that doctors make too much money.

The pollsters also asked what a fair income would be for physicians. Those polled said, oh, about $80,000 a year would be OK.

How generous. How sporting. How stupid.

Why is this poll stupid? Because it is based on resentment and envy, two emotions that ran hot during the political campaign and are still simmering.

You could conduct the same kind of poll about any group that earns $100,000-plus and get the same results. Since the majority of Americans don't make those bucks, they assume that those who do are stealing it from them.

Maybe the Berlin Wall came down, but don't kid yourself, Karl Marx lives.

It's also stupid because it didn't ask key questions, such as: Do you know how much education and training it takes to become a physician?

If those polled said, no, they didn't know, then they should have been disqualified. If they gave the wrong answers, they should have been dropped. What good are their views on how much a doctor should earn if they don't know what it takes to become a doctor?

Hard Work

Or maybe a question should have been phrased this way: "How much should a person earn if he or she must [a] get excellent grades and a fine educational foundation in high school in order to [b] be accepted by a good college and spend four years taking courses heavy in math, physics, chemistry and other lab work and maintain a 3.5 average or better, and [c] spend four more years of grinding study in medical school, with the third and fourth years in clinical training, working 80 to 100 hours a week, and [d] spend another year as a low-pay, hard-work intern, and [e] put in another three to 10 years of postgraduate training, depending on your specialty, and [f] maybe wind up $100,000 in debt after med school, and [g] then work an average of 60 hours a week, with many family doctors putting in 70 hours or more until they retire or fall over?"

As you have probably guessed by now, I have considerably more respect for doctors than does the law firm of Clinton and Clinton, and all the lawyers and insurance executives they have called together to remake America's health care.

Based on what doctors contribute to society, they are far more useful than the power-happy, ego-tripping, program-spewing, so-cial tinkerers who will probably give us a medical plan that is to health what Clinton's first budget is to frugality.

But propaganda works. And, as the stupid poll indicates, many Americans wrongly believe that profiteering doctors are the major cause of high medical costs.

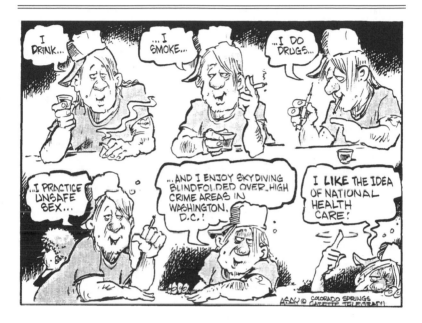

Chuck Asay, by permission of the *Colorado Springs Gazette Telegraph*.

Of course doctors are well-compensated. They should be. Americans now live longer than ever. But who is responsible for our longevity—lawyers, Congress, or the guy flipping burgers in a McDonald's?

And the doctors prolong our lives despite our having become a nation of self-indulgent, lard-butted, TV-gaping couch cabbages.

Too Many Vices

Ah, that is not something you heard President Clinton or Super Spouse talk about during the campaign or since. But in-stead of trying to turn the medical profession into a villain, they might have been more honest if they had said:

"Let us talk about medical care and one of the biggest prob-lems we have. That problem is you, my fellow American. Yes, you, eating too much and eating the wrong foods; many of you guzzling too much hooch; still puffing away at $2.50 a pack; getting your daily exercise by lumbering from the fridge to the microwave to the couch; doing dope and bringing crack babies into the world; filling the big-city emergency rooms with gunshot victims; engaging in unsafe sex and catching a deadly disease while blaming the world for not finding an instant cure.

"You and your habits, not the doctors, are the single biggest health problem in this country. If anything, it is amazing that the docs keep you alive as long as they do. In fact, I don't understand how they can stand looking at your blubbery bods all day.

"So as your president, I call upon you to stop whining and start living cleanly. Now I must go get myself a triple cheesygreasy with double fries. Do as I say, not as I do."

But for those who truly believe that doctors are overpaid, there is another solution: Don't use them.

That's right. You don't feel well? Then try one of those spinepoppers, needle-twirlers, or have Rev. Bubba lay his hands upon your head and declare you fit.

Or there is the do-it-yourself approach. You have chest pains? Then sit in front of a mirror, make a slit here, a slit there and pop in a couple of valves.

You're going to have a kid? Why throw your money at that overpaid sawbones, so he can buy a better car and a bigger house than you will ever have (while paying more in taxes and malpractice insurance than you will ever earn)?

Just have the kid the old-fashioned way. Squat and do it. And if they survive, you can go to the library and find a book on how to give them their shots.

By the way, has anyone ever done a poll on how much pollsters should earn?

"We clearly have a 'specialist glut.'"

The Glut of Specialist Physicians Hurts the Health Care System

Steven A. Schroeder

In the 1930s, 87 percent of all physicians were general practitioners—physicians who treated patients for a wide variety of health care problems. Today, only 30 percent of physicians are generalists and 70 percent are specialists—that is, anesthesiologists, cardiologists, and others who specialize in specific health care problems. In the following viewpoint, Steven A. Schroeder maintains that there are too many specialists and not enough generalists in medicine. This has increased health care costs and harmed the health care of Americans, he states. Schroeder, a generalist physician, is president of the Robert Wood Johnson Foundation, a philanthropic organization dedicated to improving the health care of Americans.

As you read, consider the following questions:

1. Why is American medicine biased toward specialists, in Schroeder's opinion?
2. How do other nations control the number of specialists, according to the author?
3. How can having a glut of specialists affect the quality of health care, in Schroeder's opinion?

"Medicine's Glut of 'Fighter Pilots'" by Steven A. Schroeder, *Los Angeles Times*, March 4, 1992. Reprinted with the author's permission.

During the early days of World War II, a U.S. fighter squadron was assigned the miserable duty of guarding a remote and unthreatened Bolivian tin mine. The pilots, young, eager and trained to the hilt, grew so desperate for any kind of action that they resorted to using their aircraft to hunt eagles flying among the mountain peaks around them—a highly dangerous waste of flying skill, fuel, ammunition and eagles.

Something akin to that contributes significantly to the spiraling cost of health care in this country. The fighter pilots, in this analogy, are specialist physicians with too few challenges to their hard-won skills.

No, it's not the "doctor glut" that we were warned about in the 1980s. That never materialized. We have about 20 practicing physicians per 10,000 people in the United States—slightly higher than in England, Canada and Australia but considerably lower than in Italy, Germany, France and Scandinavia.

A "Specialist" Glut

However, we clearly have a "specialist glut." Generalist physicians make up 50% to 75% of the medical cadres of other developed countries. In the United States, only 30% of physicians are generalists—even stretching the definition to include general internists and general pediatricians.

Medical academia is strongly biased in favor of specialists because this nation still harbors a powerful belief that what is new and exotic is the ultimate in medical care, and because, for all our talk of healthier lifestyles, we still expect our doctors to salvage us from the inevitable effects of our excesses and follies. And because specialists tend to use high-cost technologies, they earn more than general physicians. So doctors naturally want specialties, and the process by which U.S. specialists are created is unrestricted.

Left to follow its present course, the situation isn't likely to improve. Fewer than one-fourth of graduating U.S. medical students now intend to become primary-care physicians. That percentage has been dropping steadily for a decade.

In most countries, either a qualified regulatory body decides the number of specialist physicians or the supply is controlled by marketplace limits, such as limiting the level of government reimbursement for specialist procedures.

It is theoretically possible for the national residency review committee in each specialty to limit the number of specialists in training by decreasing the number of residency slots at a particular teaching hospital, or even eliminating whole programs. But if it does so on any ground other than program quality, it invites a federal restraint of trade investigation.

We have, as a result, exceeded the saturation point in many

major specialties. The predictable effect is an excess of expensive specialty procedures.

High Rates of Surgery

There is, for example, no correlation between the rate of coronary artery disease and the frequency of bypass surgery in developed countries. But there is a strong correlation between the frequency of that surgery and a nation's investment in doctors and technology to perform it. The United States has the world's highest per-capita investment in cardiac surgeons, cardiologists, catheterization labs and cardiac operating suites, and a frequency of coronary bypass surgery to match. There are similar patterns for other high-technology services like diagnostic imaging, neurosurgery, treatment of end-stage renal disease and cancer chemotherapy.

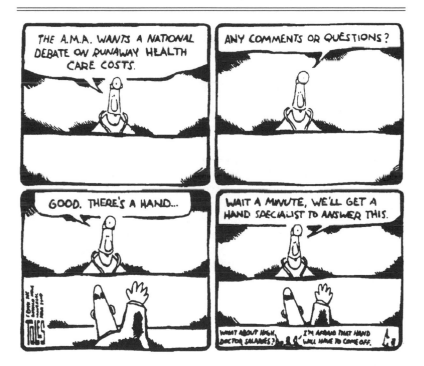

While no one can say absolutely what constitutes the "right" number of procedures, there is persuasive evidence that anywhere from 20% to 50% of the commonly performed specialty procedures in this country could be avoided without harming the health of the public.

The economic impact of such overperformance is immense. The $30,000 it costs to perform one unnecessary bypass operation would pay the annual salaries of two badly needed full-time home health aides.

The oversupply of specialists can even reduce the quality of care if patient volume falls below the level needed to maintain a specialist's technical skills. There is also increasing evidence that underemployed specialists who are obliged to practice more general medicine tend to provide higher-cost, lower-quality care outside their specialties.

Conversely, a nation with too few general physicians can't provide adequate access to basic health care for its citizens—though, admittedly, the problem of access is too complex to be addressed just by increasing the percentage of primary care physicians.

Improving General Physicians' Pay

There is the beginning of an effort to influence this imbalance by better compensation of general physicians under Medicare and Medicaid. That should be the first step toward a more thorough payment reform that reduces the bias in favor of high-technology specialties.

Government, which pays in large measure for the residency training of physicians through fees for their services to Medicare and Medicaid patients, should use that leverage to press for more emphasis on generalist programs. Loan forgiveness for physicians training for primary care specialties should be expanded.

Even if we could change all the requisite attitudes and programs overnight, it would be decades before the physician imbalance shifted adequately. The average physician practices for 40 years after he completes his training. Two generations will live with the choices each generation of physicians makes in choosing a specialty. All the more reason to start changing now.

VIEWPOINT

"The current attempt at glorification of the generalist will ultimately provide neither better care nor cost reduction."

There Is No Glut of Specialist Physicians

Joseph D. Wassersug

Many critics of the health care system advocate increasing the number of general physicians and decreasing the number of specialists. Joseph D. Wassersug disagrees. In the following viewpoint, Wassersug argues that specialists are a vital component of America's health care system. General physicians do not always provide the care patients need, he maintains. Decreasing the number of specialists will not reduce health care costs and will only decrease the quality of care that Americans receive. Wassersug is a retired internist who specialized in pulmonary and cardiovascular disease.

As you read, consider the following questions:

1. What does Wassersug mean by the term "gatekeeper," and what does he believe was their original purpose?
2. What is the federal government doing to increase the number of general physicians, according to the author?
3. How does the author compare the current attempt to reduce the number of specialists to a medical monopoly?

"Don't Deify the Role of Gatekeeper" by Joseph D. Wassersug, *American Medical News*, May 24-31, 1993. Reprinted with the author's permission.

Among the mechanisms for curbing the double-digit escalation of health care costs, the stationing of gatekeepers at the access points to care is gaining almost unquestioned acceptance. While the installation of gatekeepers may be sound from the bookkeepers' perspective, it presents a serious threat to good patient-oriented care. The gatekeeper concept came with the institution of the health maintenance organizations and, initially at least, no claims were made that the presence of gatekeepers improved medical care. Gatekeepers were hired for one purpose only—to limit or block access to the more costly services and specialists.

It was their job to take care of the easy medical problems unless they were convinced that these problems were beyond their skill. Since family practice generalists or nurse practitioners could be hired for lower wages than, let us say, cardiologists or rheumatologists, they were the ones stationed in the guardhouses.

Government Propaganda

Within a short time it became apparent that gatekeepers functioned as intended—they controlled costs. Now, the federal government, also anxious to curb the runaway health care expenses, is moving in to create more family practice physicians (and nurses) and trying to limit the numbers of "high-priced" specialists.

The propaganda machines are being activated. "We need more family practice physicians," the headlines shout; "Excess surgical specialists result in needless operations." Subsidies are being offered for medical students who agree to become family physicians. It seems as if the less-trained the doctor is, the more valuable he or she is.

Calling the loss of primary care physicians a "growing crisis," the Assn. of American Medical Colleges is urging medical schools to push half their graduates into family practice internships and residencies. The AAMC hopes that if their 126 constituent schools comply, the federal government will be less apt to intervene.

The federal government, on the other hand, is planning to increase the output of generalists through more compulsory measures. For example, meeting the goal of the congressionally appointed Council on Graduate Medical Education (50% generalists) by freezing medical school positions and setting up a residency slot allocation system made up of a national workforce commission and regional agencies. While medical schools are currently free to establish their own training programs, the COGME would force the schools to share planning decisions with government officials and other interested public agencies.

The COGME advocates weighting $5.2 billion in special graduate medical education funding so that primary care programs get more of it and specialty programs less. It also proposes strengthening scholarships and loans for those choosing primary care, and extending Medicare's improved reimbursements for generalists to all insurers. Organized medicine, COGME argues, must be more responsible to what it conceives as "societal needs." The government is planning prompt intervention and, by fiat, demanding compliance if the voluntary efforts are deemed inadequate.

Specialists Improve Quality of Medical Education

Medical educators, by establishing a high standard to medical education, have contributed greatly to assuring the competence of American physicians. The specialty societies through their residency review committees and their certification procedures have likewise had a significant effect. . . . [They] have set and pursued high standards of care which have served as a model.

Eli Ginzberg, *The Medical Triangle: Physicians, Politicians, and the Public*. Cambridge, MA: Harvard University Press, 1990.

Although this debate about primary care supply has been going on for over a decade, it has only recently reached a strident pitch. As far back as the mid-'70s, the University of Southern California studied various specialist groups as to which might best be suited for providing "primary care." Internists were initially chosen (or self-chosen) but, even back then, they were already divided into a multitude of subspecialties.

An effort is being made to glorify the gatekeeper, to applaud that role as one of "superdoc." In the *New England Journal of Medicine*, argument was advanced that gatekeepers further good medical practice because they protect "patients from the detrimental effects of unnecessary medical services."

This argument is so specious that it is not worth debating. Yet many physicians did respond. One wrote: "The gatekeeper has a tremendous financial incentive to underuse resources." Another physician cited a case from his own experience of flagrant undertreatment in an HMO [Health Maintenance Organization]. In response to this criticism, the authors of the *NEJM* essay are forced to concede that "there is a risk of undertreatment in HMOs."

Limiting the Number of Specialists

The current attempt at glorification of the generalist will ultimately provide neither better care nor cost reduction. Limitation of specialists means that in some communities there will only be one neurologist, one cardiologist, one urologist. History shows that monopolies, whether business, professional or economic, are costly and autocratic. The health of any community can be better served by diversity and challenge. Curiously, it is the policy of the federal government to view most other monopolies as restraint of trade and to deal harshly with them.

Restricting specialists means diminishing the opportunities for teaching. This is bad for both the medical schools and the students. Medical education should be in the hands of those with the greater skills, not those minimally trained.

It is disheartening to witness efforts to deify the gatekeeper. Gatekeepers may be able to play a role in controlling some of the cost of medical care, but, please, let's not glorify this role.

Periodical Bibliography

The following articles have been selected to supplement the diverse views presented in this chapter.

Sam Brody — "We Have Lost Our Humanity," *Newsweek,* September 7, 1992.

Bill Clinton — "U.S. Health Care System: Rampant Medical Inflation," *Vital Speeches of the Day,* October 15, 1993.

Hillary Rodham Clinton — "Health Care: We Can Make a Difference," *Vital Speeches of the Day,* July 15, 1993.

Sara Collins — "Desperate for Doctors," *U.S. News & World Report,* September 20, 1993.

Michael Dolan — "Cardiologist Arrest," *The Washington Monthly,* December 1992.

Christopher Georges — "Scalpel, Please," *The Washington Monthly,* September 1993.

Christine Gorman — "Is Health Care Too Specialized?" *Time,* September 14, 1992.

David A. Kindig — "The Elusive Generalist Physician," *Journal of the American Medical Association,* September 1, 1993. Available from Subscriber Services Center, American Medical Association, 515 N. State St., Chicago, IL 60610.

Melvin Konner — "We Are Not the Enemy: A Medical Opinion," *Newsweek,* April 5, 1993.

Marc L. Rivo — "Improving Access to Health Care Through Physician Workforce Reform," *Journal of the American Medical Association,* September 1, 1993.

Nina Sandlin — "Are There Too Many Doctors? And Too Many Specialists?" *American Medical News,* January 4, 1993. Available from 515 N. State St., Chicago, IL 60610.

Harry Schwartz — "Doctors' Pay a Far Cry from Athletes' Salaries: 'Ordinary' vs. 'Mythic' People to the Public," *American Medical News,* December 28, 1990.

H. Gilbert Welch — "Let's Make a Deal: Negotiating a Settlement Between Physicians and Society," *The New England Journal of Medicine,* October 29, 1992. Available from the Massachusetts Medical Society, 1440 Main St., Waltham, MA 02254.

Is Alternative
Medicine Safe?

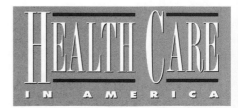

Chapter Preface

In 1983 writer Eugene Linden injured his knee in a wind-surfing accident. His physician took X rays and suggested surgery. Linden instead visited an acupuncturist. After a forty-minute session, the pain and swelling in Linden's knee was gone. He never needed the surgery.

Like Linden, many Americans are choosing alternative treatments—ranging from chiropractic medicine to acupuncture to therapy with herbs and aromas—for their health care needs. According to a 1993 study in the *New England Journal of Medicine*, in 1990 about one-third of Americans spent $10.3 billion on alternative methods.

Alternative medicine has increased in popularity for several reasons. Some Americans suffer from chronic ailments that traditional methods fail to treat effectively. Others, dissatisfied with physicians who lack the time or desire to listen to patients' problems and needs, find that practitioners of alternative medicine are more attentive and involved and often less rushed. Because alternative treatments help ease the pain of numerous Americans, many critics of the health care system applaud the growing acceptance of these treatments. "Alternative therapies should be the treatment of choice for the chronic, irritating, uninteresting maladies that plague most of us," maintains Adriane Fugh-Berman, a physician who practices alternative medicine.

Some mainstream physicians such as Fugh-Berman are using alternative methods or referring their patients to chiropractors, acupuncturists, and other nontraditional practitioners. Other physicians, however, warn that patients must exercise caution if they choose alternative methods. Herbal therapies, for example, can be lethal if misused. The government does not regulate most alternative practices, so it can be difficult to separate qualified practitioners from charlatans and to know which alternative medicines may be harmful. Finally, critics such as physician Joseph D. Wassersug argue that, while alternative practitioners may be more caring, some may not have the education or expertise to effectively treat serious illness or injury.

The controversy over the need for and effectiveness of alternative medicine will only increase as more Americans seek out such treatments. In the following chapter, the authors present their views on the value of alternative medicine.

"Using a combination of acupuncture, homeopathic medicine, and folk remedies, we've all but eliminated antibiotics from our lives. "

Alternative Medicine Can Be Safe and Effective

Sara Solovitch

In the following viewpoint, Sara Solovitch describes how her family, plagued by chronic ailments, gained relief through alternative medicine methods such as acupuncture and homeopathy. She concludes that such methods can be safe and effective, and should be used by more Americans. Solovitch is a former reporter for the *Philadelphia Inquirer* and is now a freelance writer in Santa Cruz, California, whose articles have been published in the *Washington Post, Omni,* and *The New Age Journal.*

As you read, consider the following questions:

1. How has Solovitch's pediatrician reacted to her use of alternative medicine?
2. What specific ailments of her family members have been cured through alternative medicine, according to the author?
3. How has acupuncture helped the author's family?

"Good-Bye, Antibiotics" by Sara Solovitch, *New Age Journal*, January/February 1992. Reprinted with permission.

When our first child, Ben, was born, my husband and I were as conservative about his health as any jittery new parents. We did everything according to strict Western medical dogma. The word of our pediatrician was gospel. As a consequence, Ben, who was plagued by earaches, lived on antibiotics, had the obligatory tubes put in his ears (twice), and saw the pediatrician more routinely than he did some of his friends.

By age five he was referring to his ears with unbridled loathing. "Why me?" he would wail whenever the familiar ache returned. (Interpretation: "Why not my little brother?")

Then, one day four years ago, a chance conversation with a retired physician started me thinking. The doctor said that when he had been a resident in a major Boston teaching hospital four decades ago, he rarely saw ear infections. And when he did, there wasn't even a need to look inside the ear because the symptoms were so obvious. The lobe would be red as a beet, the child screaming in agony. This doctor wondered whether the national program of vaccinations had played a role in the current epidemic of *otitis media*.

I wasn't ready to give up on vaccinations. But, finally, after years of asking why the tubes and antibiotics weren't getting the job done—and being met with the blank stares of clinicians—I was heartened to find a medical professional who was at least willing to entertain my questions. As it turned out, the retired doctor was a homeopath, a term that meant little to me at the time. All I knew was that I liked his thinking.

Nothing to Lose

A few months later, our family moved to California and found ourselves in a town where every other storefront advertised herbs, acupuncture, colon cleansers, and freshly squeezed wheat juice. We also found ourselves with a new health insurance plan that reimbursed chiropractors, homeopaths, naturopaths, and acupuncturists. So, remembering my earlier conversation with the homeopathic physician in Philadelphia, we called one when Ben came down with his next, inevitable infection. After years of frustration with the limitations of antibiotics in treating Ben's ongoing earaches, what did we have to lose—especially since the homeopath was also an M.D.?

Within fifteen minutes of taking those first tiny pellets of pulsatilla (a remedy derived from a wildflower), Ben's pain disappeared. A quick examination of his ears the next day confirmed that the infection, too, had bit the dust.

Our approach to family health hasn't been the same since. Today, using a combination of acupuncture, homeopathic medicine, and folk remedies, we've all but eliminated antibiotics from our lives. I have come to see that medicine is not the exclusive domain of doctors. Besides having my children (occasionally) enjoy my own cooking, I can't think of anything that gives me greater satisfaction than treating them successfully for simple, everyday illnesses with herbs and home remedies.

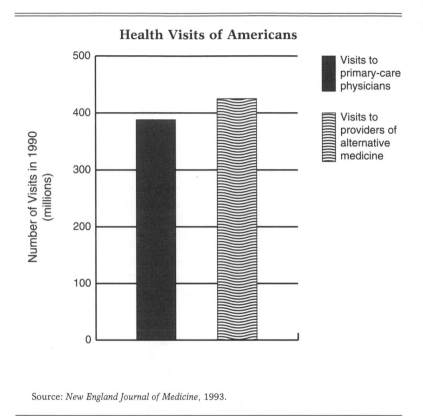

Health Visits of Americans

Source: *New England Journal of Medicine*, 1993.

My family still has a good relationship with a pediatrician —who understands and accepts his role as a back-up physician. He knows that if one of the children were seriously ill with a high fever and not responding immediately to alternative care, I wouldn't hesitate to wake him at four in the morning. And despite his occasional skepticism of our approach to family health—I've caught him rolling his eyes at the mention of some of my cures—I know that his own wife's asthma has been tremendously improved through acupuncture.

So when Ben, now eleven, gets an ear infection, I sometimes grate an onion. This remedy, I'm told, comes from India, and we have come to rely on it at three in the morning—the usual hour when Ben discovers that his ear is aching. The recipe is simple: Grate one medium onion in a blender, wrap it in a dish-cloth, and place it over the affected ear. Yes, the bedroom will reek for days, and Ben hates the smell, but he loves the relief it usually brings.

Ben's once-frequent bouts of impetigo used to mean rushing him to the pediatrician's office for a ten-day supply of penicillin. The medication would eventually relieve the ugly red blisters that spread with alarming speed around the edges of his mouth. But echinacea causes the infection to dry up even more quickly. Now, at the first signs of impetigo, I squeeze a few drops of this herbal tincture into Ben's apple juice. The infection dries up days earlier than it would with antibiotics.

Now the whole family reaches for homeopathic remedies for simple complaints that might otherwise have sent us to the drugstore. So when one of my kids is stung by a bee, I give him apis—a homeopathic remedy derived from a bee's body. When my husband, Richard, throws out his arm playing tennis, I rub a topical ointment of arnica into his shoulder. And when I have a headache, I reach for the belladonna.

A Cure with Acupuncture

To learn more about how best to treat my family, I'm taking a series of homeopathic workshops. The workshops have also taught me the sometimes fine distinctions between an ear infection calling for treatment with belladonna or one indicating pulsatilla, chamomilla, or aconite. I give belladonna to my children when their cheeks are flushed and feverish. A belladonna infection comes on somewhat more slowly than an aconite infection, which is preceded by thirst and exposure to wind. Chamomilla comes in handy when the kids are irritable, and if the pain worsens when I apply local heat to the ear. More advice is available on the remedies' labels, and through such guidebooks as the simple *Everyone's Guide to Homeopathic Remedies*, by Dana Ullman or the well-advanced *Materia Medica*, the homeopath's thick—and sometimes obscure—bible.

For some conditions we seek the advice of our acupuncturist, Martha. When Max was three years old he suffered three bouts of pneumonia in as many months—and was treated with three back-to-back rounds of antibiotics. Although Max never wheezed, his frequent colds were turning into pneumonia before the mucus had a chance to turn from clear to green.

Several doctors diagnosed the underlying problem as asthma. Their advice was to pump him up with asthma medicine at the first stage of a cold. Instead, I took him to the acupuncturist, who began a course of Chinese herbs and needles. And indeed, Max was immediately cured and hasn't had pneumonia since. (When acupuncture and homeopathy work, their effectiveness is so rapid I don't feel that there is any significant time loss that would dangerously delay seeking more help from Western medicine.)

I also called the acupuncturist once in terror, convinced that Max's red-streaked bowel movements signaled cancer. She calmly asked me—as any experienced pediatrician probably would—if he'd been eating beets. He had.

But it's not all just old-fashioned common sense. Martha wants to see the children just before the full moon each month—when their *chi*, or life force, is at its peak. And sometimes she dangles a crystal over the various vials of herbs to verify her choice of treatment. To me, with all my years of left-brain training, that still seems a little weird.

But she regularly—and instantly—cures Ben's ear infections, easily treats Max's occasional relapses of bronchitis, and once plunged me into labor when I was nearly two weeks overdue for childbirth and going out of my mind.

Unpleasant Medicine

Another time, when Jesse was sick with a respiratory illness, Martha sent us home with a repulsive-looking bag of herbs that included the molted skins of a large beetlelike insect. We brewed the substance into a tea and fed it to Jesse, then all of three months old, with an eye dropper. He didn't seem to mind, and the potion did the trick.

But, like everything else, homeopathy gets harder as the kids get older. The herbs smell awful and taste just as bad. Ben immediately knows when we've been to see Martha, and sometimes he actually refuses to get into the car because of the stench of the herbs. But he's the first one to let Martha bleed his fingers when he has an ear infection. (Finger bleeding, a practice central to classical Chinese medicine, is said to release the chi—and the blood—ultimately stimulating the body's own healing mechanisms.)

When Max occasionally must have his fingers bled, Ben urges him on: "It only hurts for a minute, Max. You know you're going to feel better as soon as it's done." Very true, but it still hurts.

A friend of ours, aware of what Ben was about to undergo, once asked: "What's next? Leeches?"

Not quite. But I've read that they are making a comeback in modern medicine. And our kids have never been healthier.

> *"My unfortunate experience has taught me that blind trust . . . is not a replacement for using common sense."*

Alternative Medicine Can Be Dangerous and Ineffective

Carolyn Copeland

Carolyn Copeland, the author of the following viewpoint, believed in and trusted her physician, who practiced alternative medicine. Ultimately though, she says, her trust threatened her life. In the viewpoint she describes her experiences with alternative medicine and warns others not to blindly trust those who practice alternative medicine. Copeland is a housewife and freelance writer in Arizona who works to inform the public about holistic health care abuses.

As you read, consider the following questions:

1. Why was Copeland initially impressed by Dr. Berry?
2. What unusual steps did the author's physician recommend?
3. What steps did the author take against Dr. Berry and Nurse Miller?

"Deception at a New Age Clinic" by Carolyn Copeland, *Vibrant Life*, July/August 1991. Reprinted by permission of the author and Review and Herald Publishing Company.

"Cancer?" I echoed disbelievingly, questioning the gynecologist's suspicion. How could I have cancer? Hadn't I followed all the instructions of Dr. James Berry [a pseudonym] and his nurse practitioner? I had practiced preventative medicine as he advised, refraining from smoking and drinking. I had yearly pelvic exams and Pap smears at his clinic.

Yet now a doctor I had never seen before was telling me I needed immediate surgery, a total hysterectomy. "If it's cancer, you don't want to wait," he urged. Whom should I trust? This gynecologist, or the health practitioners in the clinic where I had gone for 16 years?

Back in 1965 I called the county medical association and asked for the name of a general practitioner in my area. The association's telephone referral service recommended Dr. Berry. After entering the comfortable, crowded medical clinic waiting room, I was pleased to learn that my new doctor treated the whole person—body, mind, and spirit.

Dr. Berry said he believed in allowing the body to heal itself through natural processes. He and the other doctors in the clinic believed prescription drugs often produced dangerous, unwanted side effects: they prescribed them only when absolutely necessary. I was convinced illness could be averted by the commonsense methods he suggested. I thought my new doctor was wonderful! His recommendations seemed like good medical advice, dispensed by a caring physician.

Consulting the Stars

I asked Dr. Berry for help with an infertility problem and abdominal pain. He said my pelvic exam and Pap smear were normal. Then, rather than referring me to a gynecologist for further evaluation, he suggested that my husband and I have our astrological charts read to determine if we were capable of conceiving a child together.

Startled by this unorthodox approach to conception, I laughed, saying, "Our church doesn't believe in astrology."

Dr. Berry reproved me. "Don't scoff at things you don't understand."

I felt he was entitled to his beliefs about the stars, even if I didn't share them. I was consulting him for his medical expertise. His suggestion seemed unusual. But I thought, the county medical association recommended him. Surely, they wouldn't send me to a quack!

Although my husband and I never went to the astrology center, Dr. Berry instructed my husband to drink an herbal tea made with watermelon seeds to increase his sperm activity. After one "awful tasting" cupful, he refused further potions.

My abdominal pain during menses had been increasing in

severity over several years. Dr. Berry recommended castor oil packs applied to the abdomen with a heating pad, to "rid the body of accumulated wastes and poisons."

I followed his orders religiously. Each month the pain disappeared—only to return the following month. Later I learned that heat alone is an effective treatment for relieving menstrual cramps.

Alternative or Negligent Treatment?

Once I asked Dr. Berry if a cyst tumor might be causing the pain and preventing pregnancy. Soon afterward, during a pelvic exam, he found what he thought was "a small ovarian water cyst." He recommended acupuncture and performed the treatment that day in his office.

That was in 1973. Acupuncture was just gaining popularity in the United States, so I knew little about it. In time the pain recurred, and I was told to resume the castor oil pack treatment. At subsequent annual pelvic exams, Dr. Berry reassured me there was no recurrence of the cyst, even though the pain persisted.

A Last Resort

There was a time when we treated almost all major illnesses in a holistic fashion. We treated tuberculosis with fresh air and Adirondack chairs because we had not yet discovered isoniazid and streptomycin. We treated polio with Hubbard tubs and Sister Kenney physiotherapy before the advent of polio vaccines. We treated rheumatic fever with good nutrition and bed rest before there was penicillin.

Holistic medicine, it seemed to me, is what we practice when we don't know the real answer.

Joseph D. Wassersug, *American Medical News*, July 22, 1991.

In 1978 Betty Miller [a pseudonym], a family nurse practitioner, began seeing me, so I rarely saw Dr. Berry. He said Nurse Miller was almost as qualified to treat me as a doctor was, and that she could better relate to my problems from a woman's point of view. If I had any serious problems, she would consult one of the doctors.

When constipation began to plague me during my menses, Nurse Miller recommended large doses of a mild laxative, stating it wouldn't harm me because it contained "only natural ingredients." She said, "Take one teaspoonful every hour until you have a bowel movement." One time I took 17 spoonfuls.

Once during a particularly painful menstrual period, Nurse

Miller noted that I might have an ovarian cyst. Still, there was no referral to a gynecologist, so I assumed the "suspected cyst" was a false alarm. At subsequent gynecological exams, she again told me everything was "normal."

I wasn't getting any effective remedy for my abdominal pain, but I was, I thought, receiving helpful treatment for a "stubborn case" of iron-deficiency anemia. "Your body is out of balance," Dr. Berry had said in 1975. Although opposed to prescribing "dangerous prescription drugs," over-the-counter iron tablets were prescribed for me—in ever-increasing amounts as the anemia failed to respond.

Eventually Nurse Miller ordered weekly "liver and iron" shots; then she added vitamin B_{12} to the weekly injections. In addition, I was taking three 200-milligram tablets of iron every day. (Later I learned that the normal therapeutic dose is only 200 milligrams daily.) At various times they ordered other vitamins and minerals, including 1,500 milligrams of vitamin C.

Dr. Berry had also diagnosed low thyroid activity and prescribed Atomidine, a drug that could be obtained only from the clinic. Later Nurse Miller ordered a prescription thyroid medication. Little did I realize that the photomotogram they were using is an outdated measuring device, no longer considered reliable for evaluating thyroid functions.

Instead of feeling better, I felt increasingly worse—like a spaced-out zombie.

Searching for Answers

Finally in 1981 I decided to help myself by going to the library to learn more about anemia. And I decided to consult a hematologist on my own. By then I was close to physical collapse from iron and vitamin poisoning, complicated by the thyroid medication overdose. The hematologist looked at the blood counts furnished by Dr. Berry and said that I never had iron-deficiency anemia.

A bone marrow test showed that my body was satisfactorily producing red blood cells. The hematologist advised me to discontinue taking all medicine, including all vitamins.

And, on the basis of my other symptoms, he suggested I see a gynecologist. Since Nurse Miller had performed a pelvic exam just three months before and assured me everything was "normal," I was reluctant to incur the added expense of an unnecessary exam. The nurse had thoroughly convinced me there was no gynecological problem that time and menopause would not heal.

But in 1982, when I had another severe attack of abdominal pain, my hematologist insisted I see a gynecologist at once. He even made the appointment for me.

That first visit to the gynecologist was when I learned I might have cancer. The pelvic exam revealed a large mass on my left ovary. He ordered an ultrasound and kidney and liver scans, then recommended that I have surgery as soon as possible.

Two and a half weeks later, a grapefruit-sized, blood-filled cyst was removed. The gynecologist said that if the cyst had ruptured, which it could have at any time, I probably would have died. I thanked God for sparing my life.

The surgery was performed nine years after Dr. Berry first suspected an ovarian cyst and treated me with acupuncture. The cyst was pinching off the left ureter and obstructing the bowel, causing the constipation problems.

The surgeon also found both fallopian tubes obstructed with endometriosis. Had the condition been diagnosed and treated earlier, it might have been corrected. Now all my useless reproductive organs were removed, along with the cyst—and my hopes for motherhood.

Appealing for Public Protection

Holistic health care emphasizes caring and human contact—a warm, personal touch as opposed to a cold, clinical approach. My holistic healers always displayed a polished bedside manner. They were compassionate listeners, sympathetic to my every complaint and unhurried in consultation. But I also expected to receive expert medical advice and treatment.

I trusted Dr. Berry and Nurse Miller, believing that if I needed more medical attention, they would initiate a referral. The only referral they made was to an astrology center. I filed a complaint about Nurse Miller with the Arizona State Board of Nursing. Unfortunately, she is still practicing nursing, and Dr. Berry is still practicing medicine; however, the county medical referral service is no longer referring patients to him. We tend to trust people who have *M.D.* or *R.N.* behind their name. In most cases they will give us competent health care. But my unfortunate experience has taught me that blind trust of medical degrees is not a replacement for using common sense.

"Alternative approaches . . . should once again be considered as members of the family of official medicine."

Alternative Medicine Should Be Considered Standard Medical Practice

James S. Gordon

James S. Gordon, a psychiatrist, is director of the Center for Mind-Body Studies in Washington, D.C., and clinical professor in the departments of psychiatry and community and family medicine at Georgetown Medical School. In the following viewpoint, he suggests that alternative medicine practices such as herbalism and acupuncture should be incorporated into America's standard medical practices. These methods, Gordon argues, would help prevent disease, would increase patients' involvement in their own treatment, and would improve patient-physician relationships.

As you read, consider the following questions:

1. What criticisms does Gordon have of how modern medicine treats disease?
2. What does the author mean by "self-regulation," and how does it work?
3. What can Americans learn from indigenous cultures, according to Gordon?

"Taking a Holistic Approach to Health Care Reform" by James S. Gordon, *The Washington Post National Weekly Edition*, September 6-12, 1993. Reprinted with the author's permission.

The long-term success of health care reform depends on the creation of a collaborative and respectful physician-patient partnership. It requires a profound shift in emphasis from authoritarian medical intervention to authoritative self-care. Much of what we have tended to regard as peripheral or trivial must become central: the therapeutic use of nutrition, exercise and relaxation; the mobilization of the mind to alter and transform itself and the body; group support. Techniques that are fundamental to the healing systems of other cultures—such as acupuncture and yoga—should be fully integrated into our own. Alternative approaches, nourished on our own soil yet largely scorned by the medical establishment—herbalism, chiropractic and prayer among them—should once again be considered as members of the family of official medicine.

This open-minded, integrated approach grows out of a sense of the origins and dimensions of our present health care crisis. It in turn must be predicated on profound changes in the kind of care we pay for: our research priorities and our medical education. The key is understanding what we have lost as well as gained through our high-tech, disease-oriented medicine.

Focus on Chronic Diseases

Over the past 75 years, the burden of disease in the United States has changed from acute, life-threatening emergencies to chronic, often stress-related illnesses. These maladies range from arthritis and cardiovascular disease to cancer, depression and AIDS. The toll that chronic illness takes increases each year, and each year it is generally disproportionately greater for the poor and, in particular, for people of color. All may be shaped by the ways we think and feel, eat and exercise, work and play, by our economy, our environment and our interpersonal world.

The surgical and pharmacological remedies that modern biomedicine has developed are potent and effective in emergencies, but for most chronic illness they are little more than palliative. And all too often, both surgical and pharmacological treatments are used inappropriately, produce significant and deleterious side effects and are overpriced.

As things now stand, neither those who receive nor those who provide health care are satisfied with the results. A 1991 American Medical Association survey noted that 69 percent of those polled believed that "people are beginning to lose faith in doctors" and that 63 percent felt that "doctors are too interested in making money." Some physicians are not happy either. A poll done by the AMA in 1989 indicated that as many as one-quarter of those who are currently in practice "probably would not go" to medical school if they had it to do over.

Both patients and their doctors are frustrated by the lack of con-

107

tinuity in their relationships, by delays and by the impersonality of contact. In even the best of relationships, patients are troubled by their physicians' inability to address either the biological or the psychosocial dimensions of chronic, stress-related problems.

Looking for a New Approach to Health

The growth of alternative medicine, now a $27 billion-a-year industry, is more than just an American flirtation with exotic New Age thinking. It reflects a gnawing dissatisfaction with conventional, or "allopathic," medicine. For all its brilliant achievements—the polio vaccine, penicillin, transplant surgery—conventional medicine, many folks feel, has some serious weak spots, not the least of which is the endless waiting in paper gowns for doctors who view you as a sore back, an inoperable tumor or a cardiac case rather than a person. . . . Says Dr. Stephan Rechtschaffen, an M.D. who uses a preventive approach to healing: . . . "People are fed up with the old answers. They are beginning to realize that illness does not just drop out of the sky and hit them over the head. Health is an ongoing process."

Claudia Wallis, *Time*, November 4, 1991.

As we've started to perceive the limits of surgical and pharmacological interventions, we've also begun to appreciate the benefits of efforts we can make on our own behalf. The 1988 surgeon general's report "Research on Nutrition" makes clear the contribution of poor nutrition—in particular, diets high in animal fat and refined sugar and low in fiber—to cardiovascular disease, strokes and cancer, as well as to diabetes and digestive disorders. Studies on various kinds of physical exercise have demonstrated substantial physiological and psychological improvement as a consequence of regular activity.

The potential of the mind to directly affect the body is even more striking. The capacity for self-regulation that once seemed unbelievable even in Indian yogis is now commonplace in our clinics. Biofeedback, relaxation and simple visual images may enable us to change our heart rate, blood flow, urine output, brain-wave patterns and even the numbers and activity of white blood cells, often with demonstrable clinical benefits.

A New Perspective

In the past 25 years we have also begun to rediscover the healing traditions of other cultures and long-neglected Western therapeutic systems. For example, acupuncture conceives of mind and body as inseparable and postulates a continuous and animating flow of Qi, or energy. It has repeatedly been shown to release mood-altering and pain-relieving endorphins, to decrease chronic pain, to reduce the craving of addicts and alcoholics and to improve mood in depressed people.

It has become clear too that the effect of any therapeutic interventions—conventional or alternative, Western or non-Western—may be enhanced by loving, individual attention from health care providers and group support from others with similar illnesses. This is true at every stage of life and in virtually every chronic illness.

Taken together, these shifts are providing the basis for a new vision of medicine. We haven't yet agreed on a name for it, but we do know this medicine when we practice it or share its results with our colleagues. Our patients know it too. Witness the extraordinary popularity of the Bill Moyers series, "Healing and the Mind." An article by David Eisenberg and his colleagues in the *New England Journal of Medicine* revealed that as many as 34 percent of adult Americans had used "alternative therapies" in a single year.

If we are to address the causes as well as the symptoms of our health care crisis—if we are to provide not just basic coverage but genuine service—we need to learn some fundamental lessons:

• *Creating healing partnerships.* Compliance with "doctor's orders" is based on domination and often produces distance and antagonism. Collaboration is grounded in shared information, full patient participation and, most importantly, the physician's respect for a patient's capacity to understand his situation and its alternatives, and then to make the choices that make sense. This more democratic relationship shifts some of the responsibility for health care to patients and allows them to reap the additional psychological and physiological rewards of feeling more in control of their own lives.

• *Making self-care primary care.* Medicine recognizes self-care as useful—women are routinely instructed to examine their breasts—but we have only recently begun to explore its range and power. Some of the most dramatic results in the treatment of major illnesses have been obtained by teaching patients self-help in the context of sustained group support.

Treating Heart Disease

Dean Ornish and his colleagues at the Preventive Medicine Research Institute have demonstrated that "comprehensive lifestyle changes"—including a one-year program of low-fat vegetarian diets, cessation of smoking, stress management training, yoga, meditation and moderate exercise—can produce dramatic improvements in cardiac functioning in patients with serious coronary artery disease. In a 10-year follow-up study of women with metastatic breast cancer published in 1989, Stanford

University psychiatrist David Spiegel showed that women who participated in a group that used mutual support, self-hypnosis and guided imagery lived, on average, 18 months longer than those in a control group.

• *Examining alternative medicines.* Informed curiosity about the nonconventional approaches that so many people find useful should be second nature to health care professionals who are genuinely concerned with their patients' well being. Overcoming the narrowness of our bias will have many benefits. It will help promote more humility in physicians and improve our communication with the 70 percent of our patients who, according to Eisenberg's study, never discuss the alternative therapies they use with their doctors.

• *Restructuring financing.* Our current reimbursement system rewards diagnostic and surgical procedures at 10, 20—even 50—times the rate of equivalent amounts of time spent listening to, educating and counseling patients. To redress this imbalance, we should give talking, teaching and prevention as high an economic priority as technological treatment. At the same time, we need to do radical surgery on a malpractice system that frightens physicians into gross overuse of these tests and procedures.

We also need to use reimbursement guidelines to encourage approaches that maximize self-care and mutual support and minimize the use of invasive procedures and prescribed medication. In 1990, for example, about 285,000 angioplasties and 392,000 bypass surgeries were performed on cardiac patients. The average cost of an angioplasty (a procedure that uses a balloon to expand arteries) for people under 65 was about $14,000; for bypass surgery, $43,000. Many of these people closely resemble (in age and illness) those who successfully participated in Dean Ornish's year-long educational program. In Ornish's study, the heart patients saw improvements at a cost of $3,500 to $4,000 per person.

Achieving Balance

• *Reallocating research priorities.* We need a research agenda that reflects both the practical and conceptual concerns of the patient-centered care we are creating. Some of the studies will be traditional in form if innovative in content—for example, investigating the anatomical and physiological bases and clinical efficacy of approaches such as chiropractic and acupuncture, from which millions of Americans seek help.

• *Understanding illness as a transformative process and the healer's work as a sacred trust.* In many indigenous cultures illness is understood as a sign of imbalance between the individual and the social, natural and spiritual world as well as imbalance within the individual. This understanding helps make illness intelligible to the patient, gives larger meaning to his or her suffering. It also provides the rationale for future changes in behavior and attitude.

If we modern healers wish to perform the same service for our patients, we must first explore our own blind spots. We must fashion a new kind—and also a very old kind—of deeply personal medical education for ourselves and for those who come after us.

Only those who are exposed to the healing systems of other cultures and times will have a critical perspective on our own medicine. Only physicians who are taught to temper the arrogance that inevitably comes with status and expertise with the humbling power of self-awareness can heal themselves and teach others to do likewise.

"The main reason for quackery's success is its ability to seduce people who are unsuspecting or desperate."

Alternative Medicine Should Not Be Considered Standard Medical Practice

Stephen Barrett

Most alternative medicine is dangerous quackery, Stephen Barrett contends in the following viewpoint. He charges that media reports portray alternative practices positively, leading Americans to believe such practices are safe and beneficial. Unfortunately, he concludes, alternative medicine poses a threat to public health and consequently should not be incorporated into standard medical practice. Barrett, a psychiatrist and consumer advocate, edits *Nutrition Forum Newsletter* and has written and edited numerous books.

As you read, consider the following questions:

1. How are claims concerning the effectiveness of alternative practices misleading, in Barrett's opinion?
2. Why does the author oppose testing alternative methods for their effectiveness?
3. Why does Barrett believe it is unfair to blame physicians for the increased interest in alternative medicine?

Promoters of quackery are adept at using slogans and buzz-words. During the 1970s, they popularized the word "natural" as a magic sales slogan. During the 80s, the word "holistic" gained similar use. Today's leading buzzword is "alternative." Correctly employed, it refers to methods that have equal value for a particular purpose. (An example would be two antibiotics capable of killing a particular organism.) When applied to un-proven methods, however, the term can be misleading because methods that are unsafe or ineffective are not reasonable alter-natives to proven treatments. For this reason, I place the word "alternative" in quotation marks when it refers to methods that are not based on established scientific knowledge.

"Alternative" practitioners typically use anecdotes and testimo-nials to promote their practices. When someone feels better after having used a product or procedure, it is natural to credit what-ever was done. This can be misleading, however, because most ailments resolve themselves and those that persist can have vari-able symptoms. Even serious conditions can have sufficient day-to-day variation to enable quack methods to gain large followings. In addition, taking action often produces temporary relief of symptoms (a placebo effect). People who are not aware of these facts tend to give undeserved credit to "alternative" methods.

Misleading Publicity

The news media publicizes "alternative" methods in ways that can foster great public confusion. Most of their reports contain little critical thinking and feature the views of proponents and their satisfied clients. In 1992, *Time, Newsweek* and *U.S. News & World Report* published feature articles. "Good Morning America" and "CBS This Morning" aired snippets for a week, and CBS's "48 Hours" aired a one-hour show.

Many of these reports exaggerated the significance of the newly opened National Institutes of Health office for the study of uncon-ventional medical practices (now called the Office of Alternative Medicine). *Time*, for example, stated that, "The NIH program is supported by an odd alliance of New Age believers and old-school quackbusters. Both sides want to sort out once and for all what works." The article was titled, "New Age Meets Hippocrates: Medicine gets serious about unconventional therapy."

Taken together, these reports suggest that "alternative" meth-ods have become increasingly accepted by the public, even though (as I had pointed out to several reporters) no valid data exist to enable comparison of past and present utilization of most "alternative" practices.

In January 1993, the *New England Journal of Medicine* published "Unconventional Medicine in the United States," an article by David Eisenberg, M.D., and five collaborators. The report was based on a telephone survey concerning the use of 16 types of "unconventional therapy" among 1,539 individuals. The authors concluded:

In 1990 Americans made an estimated 425 million visits to providers of unconventional therapy. This number exceeds the number of visits to all U.S. primary care physicians (388 million). Expenditures . . . amounted to approximately $13.7 billion.

The study's design was extremely poor. The authors define "unconventional therapies" as "medical intervention not taught widely at U.S. medical schools or generally available at U.S. hospitals." However, the categories they selected included some approaches that are medically appropriate (self-help groups, for example) and some that may or may not be appropriate, depending on the circumstances (relaxation therapy, biofeedback, hypnosis, massage and commercial weight-loss clinics). Thus, the estimated expense total is meaningless.

The Problems with Some Alternative Methods

Acupuncture: . . . Although acupuncture can sometimes relieve pain, there is no evidence that it can influence the course of any organic disease. . . .

"Holistic" approach: . . . Most practitioners who call themselves "holistic" use unscientific methods for diagnosis and treatment. . . .

Macrobiotic diet: A semi-vegetarian diet claimed by its proponents to improve health and prolong life. Proponents suggest that the diet is effective in preventing and treating cancer, AIDS, and other serious disease. There is no evidence to support these claims.

Quackwatch, Spring 1993.

In February 1993, the Public Broadcasting System aired a five-part series called "Healing and the Mind," narrated by Bill Moyers. The topics included Chinese medicine, "the relationship between the immune system and our emotions," group therapy and meditation, "the art of healing," and treatment at Commonweal, a "retreat center for people with cancer." Dr. Eisenberg, an instructor at Harvard Medical School, was the principal consultant for the series. In an interview in *USA Today*, he said that he hoped to create a teaching center "dedicated to the rigid assessment of unconventional therapies" with "a lot of political support and a lot of money to fund and implement." When asked how our already overburdened health-care system can afford to study unconventional methods, he replied, "How can we not spend millions of dollars to understand which are safe, effective and could save money?"

The answer, of course, is that large amounts of money should not be invested in testing methods for which there is no *preliminary* evidence of effectiveness. Preliminary research does not require funding or even take much effort. The principal ingredients are careful clinical observations, detailed record keeping and long-term follow-up to "keep score." Proponents of "alternative" methods almost never do these things. Most who clamor for research do so as a ploy to arouse public sympathy—the last thing they want is a scientific test that could prove them wrong. Should scientific studies be performed and come out negative, proponents invariably claim that the studies were conducted improperly or that the evaluators were biased.

In 1991, at the urging of a former congressman who had used an "alternative" cancer therapy, Congress enacted a law ordering NIH to foster research into unconventional practices and allocating $2 million per year for two years to begin the job. Early in 1992, NIH appointed a 20-person advisory panel that included the former congressman, Dr. Eisenberg and leading advocates of acupuncture, energy medicine, homeopathy, Ayurvedic medicine and several types of "alternative" cancer therapies. A few qualified researchers were chosen for the panel, but they had little influence over subsequent events. The panel members did not have to file conflict-of-interest statements or promise to refrain from using their advisory status in advertising their products and services. In June, the panel met for two days to discuss research principles and to hear testimony from more than 50 assorted practitioners. In September, the panelists met in committees that submitted suggestions for further action. Many of the panelists have trumpeted their association with NIH as evidence that whatever "alternative" methods they promote are valid.

The NIH office is preparing to consider proposals to fund studies of several methods. It remains to be seen whether such studies will be funded and will yield useful results. Even if useful research is conducted, however, its benefit is unlikely to outweigh the publicity bonanza given to quack methods.

It is often suggested that people seek "alternatives" because doctors are brusque, and that if doctors were more attentive, their patients would not turn to quacks. Doctors sometimes pay insufficient attention to the emotional needs of their patients. But blaming the medical profession for quackery's success would be like blaming astronomers for the popularity of astrology. The main reason for quackery's success is its ability to seduce people who are unsuspecting or desperate. The massive publicity given to "alternatives" will do exactly that.

"Chiropractors . . . work with the normal functions of the human condition to assist the body's own defenses to correct illness."

Chiropractors Can Help Heal Many Ailments

Stephen J. Press and Jennifer Drawbridge

Stephen J. Press, founder and president of the International Federation of Sports Chiropractic (FICS) and secretary-general of the World Fitness Federation, has offices in Englewood, New Jersey, and Moscow, Russia. In Part I of the following viewpoint, he describes the training and work of chiropractors. In Part II of the viewpoint, Jennifer Drawbridge discusses the increasing acceptance of chiropractic by "mainstream" medicine, and cites recent studies that have found chiropractic more effective than conventional therapies for some physical problems. Drawbridge is a freelance writer who specializes in health issues.

As you read, consider the following questions:

1. What kind of education is required for a doctor of chiropractic, according to Press?
2. What effect did the AMA (American Medical Association) have on chiropractic in the past, according to the authors? Why has that situation changed?
3. Drawbridge cites studies that show that most back pain will subside with or without treatment. Why does she suggest that chiropractic treatment should be considered for such pain anyway?

Stephen J. Press, "So You're Going to a Chiropractor," *Health News & Review*, December 1991. Copyright © 1991 by Keats Publishing, Inc. Published by Keats Publishing, Inc., New Canaan, CT. Reprinted with permission. Jennifer Drawbridge, "The Chiropractic Cure: An Old Technique Is Gaining New Recognition in the Treatment of Back Pain." This article originally appeared in the April 1993 issue of *Glamour.* Reprinted with permission.

I

Before you decide whether or not to see a Doctor of Chiropractic (D.C.), you should know what they are and what they do.

A D.C. is a licensed physician, trained to diagnose diseases the same as an M.D. (allopathic physician). The schooling is approximately the same, except that the D.C. goes to chiropractic college instead of medical school. The D.C. takes national and state board exams similar to those of medicine and receives a license to practice from a state agency in any state in which he or she wishes to practice. (All 50 states license chiropractic.)

Many other countries now grant licenses as well, and most give the right to practice whatever was taught in the accredited chiropractic college. In the U.S., nearly all chiropractic institutions are accredited by the Council on Chiropractic Education (CCE), which is itself recognized by the Federal government, and the Council on Post-Secondary Accreditation (COPA). All the CCE-accredited colleges are in turn accredited by the regional agencies accrediting all the colleges and universities in the country: the Middle States Association, Southern States, etc.

Virtually all such colleges are five academic years long, and all require at least two years of college as a prerequisite (the same legal requirement as all medical schools).

Helping the Body Heal Itself

However, Doctors of Chiropractic generally study three times the anatomy and physiology of typical medical students, and this is appropriate as this type of practice depends on their thorough understanding of the normal functioning of the human body.

Chiropractors give no drugs and practice no surgery, but instead, work with the normal functions of the human condition to assist the body's own defenses to correct illness.

Can the D.C. cure cancer or heart disease? No, but the human body does suffer a wide range of disease which can be successfully resolved by the body's own capabilities—if given the chance to do so.

So what does the D.C. usually treat? Unfortunately, due to the orchestrated and illegal boycott by the AMA and organized medicine (which was proven in the federal courts in the past couple of years), the true nature of the range of services chiropractors have to offer was not widely available information. So the average new patient generally comes to the chiropractic office with some kind of backache, neck, arm, or shoulder pain or something of the kind. It's only when the patient has received adjustments found safe and effective that he or she asks more about services the chiropractor can render.

The chiropractic physician can also be your family doctor, helping you stay truly healthy through preventive maintenance. By keeping all the joints in your spine properly moving, the D.C. prevents interference with your nervous system, and allows your body's "life force" to express itself through your nerves. This is a process known to the physiologist as "homeostasis," or proper balance of life forces. Too much or too little of this or that, and your system is out of kilter.

M.D.s Can Now Work with Chiropractors

One important breakthrough came in 1991, when a federal court chastised the American Medical Association for establishing a code of ethics that prohibited M.D.s from professionally associating with chiropractors. Since the victory, M.D.s have been free to refer patients to chiropractors and to work alongside them in labs and hospitals.

There may . . . be a patient-driven trend toward more unorthodox sources of treatment, says Joseph Jacobs, M.D., director of the National Institutes of Health's newly formed Office of Alternative Medicine, an office congressionally mandated to explore untraditional therapies. Many Americans are losing confidence in medical science, Dr. Jacobs suggests, and the personalized, natural methods of alternative practitioners may reassure them.

Alice Bredin, *Mademoiselle*, May 1993.

Your nervous system controls all of these forces, and the spine is its switchboard. So such conditions as bronchial asthma, menstrual cramps, some allergies and migraine headaches (to name a few) respond well to chiropractic care.

The Athletes' Edge

More and more, the person in tune with his or her body is becoming savvy to the benefits of chiropractic adjustments. The athlete, the dancer, the performer . . . the U.S. Olympic Team officially includes a D.C. at all Olympic games. The Soviet Sport Committee sent a Western-trained D.C. to the Olympics with its teams, as many other national Olympic teams have, because the Olympic athlete needs every edge he or she can get. They can feel the difference a chiropractic adjustment provides.

Imagine the value to your body, if even an Olympic athlete can be improved by the fine-tuning the D.C. can render!

How do you choose a chiropractor? Certainly not from the phone book, except as a last resort! Ask around, get a few recommendations from friends. If no one you know is a chiropractic patient, you can check the directory, but call around. Which college did the doctor go to? Is it CCE-accredited? Is the doctor board-certified in one or more of the recognized specialties (sports, orthopedics, neurology, imaging or nutrition)? Does the doctor attend regular continuing education seminars at the college or just practice management courses? Tough questions, but you are entitled to the answers.

If all else fails, call the American Chiropractic Association in Alexandria, Virginia, to get the name of someone in your area who is a member. If you are an athlete, ask who is board-certified in sports chiropractic in your area.

II

The movers were late, and Kathy Byrnes, eager to settle into her new office, decided to move a few desks by herself. Byrnes, a fund-raiser for Health Care for All, a nonprofit organization in Boston, eventually wound up flat on her back and unable to get out of bed. When she finally managed to hobble to a doctor, he gave her a prescription for muscle relaxants and two words of advice: "Take them." Byrnes opted instead to see a chiropractor.

Although chiropractic medicine has been around for almost a century, it has only recently gained a growing, if somewhat reluctant, acceptance by mainstream medicine. The thaw in M.D.-chiropractor relations is due, at least in part, to the recent settlement of a bitter and prolonged lawsuit in which a group of chiropractors successfully argued that the American Medical Association (AMA) was conspiring to eliminate the practice of chiropractic in the U.S. The case for chiropractic has been given a further boost by recent studies suggesting that for certain kinds of back pain, chiropractic care may speed recovery faster than traditional medical care.

More than 18 million Americans visit chiropractors each year, according to a recent Gallup survey. The vast majority seek relief from back and neck pain. For many patients, including Byrnes, a big part of the attraction is the conservative chiropractic philosophy—practitioners use neither drugs nor surgery. Estelle Bolofsky, a New York City office supervisor suffering from debilitating neck pain, got cold feet when her orthopedist mentioned surgery. "When someone suggested their chiropractor, I was so desperate, I said, 'I'll do it.'"

The Case for Spinal Manipulation

Both Byrnes and Bolofsky were treated with spinal manipulation, a technique usually involving use of the hands that's the cornerstone of chiropractic therapy. "When I describe it to patients, I say it's like freeing a rusty bolt," says Daniel Futch, D.C. (Doctor of Chiropractic), chief of the chiropractic staff at Group

Health Cooperative, a Madison, Wisconsin, health-maintenance organization. "I examine the spine, looking for vertebrae that aren't moving normally. If I find one, I use a forceful movement to push it just beyond its normal range of motion, but not so far that the joint is injured." No one—chiropractors included—knows precisely how manipulation works, but it's believed that restoring mobility to a formerly fixed joint can relieve tension and pressure on adjoining muscles, joints and nerves, thereby reducing or even eliminating nagging back pain.

Studies Show Chiropractic Works

In a report released in July 1991 by the Rand Corp., a prestigious research organization in Santa Monica, Calif., a panel of leading physicians, osteopaths and chiropractors found that chiropractic-style manipulation was helpful for a major category of patients with lower-back pain: people who are generally healthy but who had developed back trouble within the preceding two or three weeks. Another important study published in the *British Medical Journal* compared chiropractic treatment with outpatient hospital care that included traction and various kinds of physical therapy. Its conclusion: spinal manipulation was more effective for relieving low-back aches for up to three years after diagnosis. . . .

By some estimates, 75% of all Americans will suffer from low-back aches at some point in their lifetime. The annual cost to U.S. society of treating the ubiquitous ailment was recently tallied at a crippling $24 billion, compared with $6 billion for AIDS and $4 billion for lung cancer. If spinal manipulation could ease even a fraction of that financial burden, remaining skeptics might be forced to stifle their misgivings or get cracking themselves.

Andrew Purvis, *Time*, September 23, 1991.

Manipulation took care of Byrnes's back pain. "I couldn't believe the noises coming from my body during my first visit," she says. (Noises result from the benign release of gases in the joints and are not harmful.) "My spine kept cracking and popping. But the treatment wasn't painful, and I felt better immediately." Bolofsky didn't hear any cracks or pops, but she, too, experienced considerable relief after just a few manipulations.

In fact, new studies indicate that many Americans might benefit from chiropractic care—specifically, the estimated 80 percent of the population who suffer from back pain at some point in their lives. For example, a 1990 *British Medical Journal* report that compared chiropractic therapy for low-back pain with more conventional hospital treatments concluded that chiropractic was more successful, particularly for patients plagued by chronic and severe pain.

A small but growing number of chiropractors, fueled by this kind of evidence, now limit their practices exclusively to muscular and skeletal disorders of the back. But many chiropractors remain loyal to one of the original tenets of chiropractic medicine, the subluxation theory, which holds that pressure on nerves from misaligned vertebrae makes the body more vulnerable to ills ranging from the common cold to heart disease.

The earliest followers of Daniel Palmer, the nineteenth-century founder of chiropractic medicine, touted manipulation as the cure-all for disease. Today's doctors of chiropractic, with the requisite six years of training, aren't that simplistic, but many do see chiropractic as an important adjunct to conventional medical treatment. By adjusting the spine, these traditional chiropractors believe that they restore proper nerve function and allow the body to return more quickly to good health. . . . There are plenty of patients who state with confidence that their headaches, allergies, depression or menstrual cramps were cured by spinal manipulation. But so far, the only chiropractic claim that's backed up by hard scientific evidence is that chiropractors can remedy sore backs and necks.

The Chiropractic Exam

A first-time chiropractic examination is not unlike most traditional medical exams, according to Louis Sportelli, D.C., former chairman of the board of the American Chiropractic Association. The chiropractor checks vital signs and takes a detailed medical history. What's different is that the chiropractic practitioner spends more time than the average medical doctor looking at posture, examining the spine and testing reflexes and joint motion in a search for clues to the patient's problem. This initial exam may take 30 minutes to an hour to complete.

At one time, chiropractors considered a full-body X ray a necessary part of a thorough first exam. However, practitioners now agree that such an X ray is of little diagnostic use and exposes the patient to an unnecessary dose of radiation. But many chiropractors continue to prescribe more limited spinal X rays for their patients. Be sure that you understand and agree with your chiropractor's X ray recommendations before you start treatment.

Among the 45,000 chiropractors in the U.S., there is a wide range of treatment methods. Treatments can take five minutes or last an hour. They can be done while patients lie down, stand up, bend, kneel or sit. They're done on special tables or chairs. The adjustments may be feather-light or forceful. However it's done, "manipulation of the low back is a very safe procedure," says Dr. Futch. "Even in the neck area, where there are arteries

vulnerable to damage, there are very few reported injuries."
While manipulation itself is usually painless (a minority of patients report some discomfort), it's not uncommon to feel achy for 12 to 24 hours after treatment.

Costs vary almost as much as therapies do; you can expect to pay from $25 to $80 a visit, depending on where you live. At least part of that tab is often reimbursed by insurance companies. Be aware, however, that the per-visit fee may not include prices for extras such as nutritional supplements or massages, which some chiropractors consider an indispensable part of therapy. If you don't want them, phone around to find a chiropractor who doesn't insist on these add-ons. . . .

Fortunately, the majority of chiropractors are frank about fees and are willing to give you their best estimate of how long therapy will take, even though it's almost impossible to predict the *exact* number of adjustments that will be needed to clear up a particular problem. Cara Lipshie, a Manhattan copywriter, was lucky: It took just one visit to a chiropractor to relieve neck pain caused by a switch in her usual swim stroke. Diane Adler, a New York City fund-raiser who went to the same chiropractor with a severe case of low-back pain, required six months of regular weekly visits to get better. Most patients fall somewhere in between these two and can expect to find relief within 6 to 12 visits.

If your back pain hasn't been significantly reduced after a few weeks of chiropractic treatment, consider looking for a second opinion from another chiropractor or an M.D. "Studies show that if chiropractic is going to work, odds are it will work within one to six weeks," says Dr. Futch. The fact is, in more than 90 percent of back-pain cases involving an uncomplicated strain, symptoms subside within 2 to 12 weeks with or *without* treatment. But chiropractic care, according to a 1992 report in the *Annals of Internal Medicine*, can speed this natural recovery process in some cases. And that can translate into fewer days of pain and fewer days of being unable to bend, lift, turn your head or tie your shoes.

"Chiropractic is still a significant hazard to many patients."

Chiropractors Can Cause Serious Injuries

George Magner

Many chiropractors contend that they can treat numerous ailments by manipulating a patient's spine. In the following viewpoint, George Magner asserts that chiropractors inflict many severe injuries, such as paralysis and nerve damage, on their patients. Magner cites physicians, consumer groups, and scientists who oppose the practice of chiropractic. Magner, who was injured by a chiropractor, is the founder of Victims of Chiropractic, an organization that works to inform the public concerning the dangers of chiropractic medicine.

As you read, consider the following questions:

1. What are some of the potential complications of spinal manipulation, according to the author?
2. What suggestions does Magner give to those concerned about chiropractic?
3. How can one find a good chiropractor, according to Magner?

From "Can You Trust Your Chiropractor?" by George Magner, a publication of Victims of Chiropractic, 1310 Union Church Rd., Watkinsville, GA 30677. Reprinted with the author's permission.

"Chiropractic is based on a false theory." [Peter J. Modde in *Legal Aspects of Medical Practice*.] . . .

"There is very little substantiated scientific evidence that any of the major things [chiropractors] do are either valid or reliable." [Jack A. Ebner in *ACA Journal of Chiropractic*.]

"Although many chiropractors firmly believe manipulating the spine can prevent or treat disease, there's no evidence it can do that." [Daniel Futch in *American Health*.] . . .

Are these the biased, uninformed statements of medical doctors supposedly in competition with chiropractors? No, they are admissions either by *chiropractors* themselves, or by academics writing in *chiropractic journals*.

Consumer Protection and Research Organizations

What do independent consumer protection and research organizations have to say about chiropractic?

"Much of what they do is unscientific or unethical."—Consumers Union.

"Overall, CU believes that chiropractic is still a significant hazard to many patients."—Consumers Union.

"NCAHF believes that a health care delivery system as confused and poorly regulated as is chiropractic constitutes a major consumer health problem."—National Council Against Health Fraud. . . .

Scientists and M.D.s

What do those who practice by the rigorous standards and safeguards of the scientific method think about chiropractic? . . .

"There is no rational basis for their theories and no objective evidence to support their sweeping claims."—Arnold Relman, M.D.

"There is no scientific evidence that manipulation is effective in the treatment of acute or chronic neck problems, and there have been a number of tragic complications associated with its use. It is the authors' feeling that the hazards are too great and that manipulation has no place in the treatment of cervical spine disorders."—Scott Boden, M.D., et al.

"Starkly put, there's no clinical or scientific evidence to suggest that manipulation can help cure systemic diseases such as diabetes, ulcers, hypertension, and so on. Anyone who knowingly or unknowingly attempts to treat such diseases with manipulation renders a great disservice to his fellow humans."—Augustus A. White III, M.D.

Deception

If most of the above is news to you, then you may have been deceived. There are numerous deceptions, such as the claim that small misalignments ("subluxations") of the spinal vertebrae can cause spinal nerve root impingement. This foundational chiropractic theory has been conclusively disproven by the work of Edmund Crelin, Ph.D. The discrediting of that classical chiropractic theory makes an irrelevant hypothesis of the claim that the supposed impingement of spinal nerves can cause visceral, systemic, and even infectious diseases. No wonder that such a preposterous claim "contradicts much of the basic medical knowledge of the twentieth century" [according to Consumers Union]. It also contradicts good common sense: If such a claim were true then people with scoliosis (lateral curvature of the spine) would have every disease on the chiropractors' fanciful

Two Thoracic Vertebrae

Do small misalignments of the spinal vertebrae cause them to impinge upon the nerve roots exiting the spinal column through the intervertebral foramina (the openings formed by notches in two adjacent vertebrae)? A prominent anatomist has conclusively proven that they cannot unless there is a force great enough to break the spine.

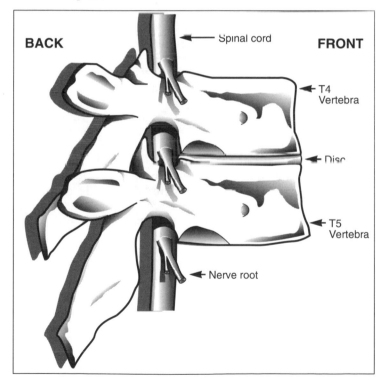

BACK ← Spinal cord FRONT

← T4 Vertebra

← Disc

← T5 Vertebra

← Nerve root

Drawing by Grafikus.

nerve charts, and quadriplegics would all be dead. If chiropractors don't believe the above claims, then what are those Parker nerve charts doing on their walls and in their literature detailing the supposed disease effects of alleged nerve impingements at the various vertebrae?

There is also the common claim that "preventive maintenance" adjustments can help prevent disease. Also scientifically disproven by Dr. Crelin's research, that spurious assertion has been well described [by Consumers Union] as a clever way to "fleece healthy people as well as sick people." These false claims work to waste your time and money primarily. The most serious deception, however, is the assurance that spinal manipulation as practiced by chiropractors is safe. This deception can work to waste your health and your very life!

Serious Risks

What exactly are the major risks? The National Chiropractic Mutual Insurance Company, a chiropractic malpractice insurer, lists the injuries (and the percentage of the total) for which they paid out claims in 1990 as: 1) Bone fractures—21%, 2) Cerebrovascular accidents [strokes]—20%, 3) Disc rupture—19%, 4) Failure to diagnose—18%, 5) Vicarious [sic, they probably mean various]—11%, 6) Soft tissue injury—8%.

Personal communication by a reformed chiropractor with the insurer ascertained that the total number of claims paid that year was about 700. Thus, taking 20 percent of 700 tells us that there were about 140 stroke claims paid out by this one company in 1990. Doubtless, this is just the tip of the iceberg since there are other chiropractic malpractice insurers. In a remarkable report the Harvard Medical Practice Study III concluded that less than 3 percent of patients experiencing adverse events caused by negligence as defined strictly ever file malpractice claims. Since the demographics of users of chiropractic services is roughly comparable to that of non-users, there is no reason to believe that the situation is any better in regard to chiropractic. It must be emphatically noted that, as opposed to chiropractic, medical science does provide reliable figures on rates of complications, and that those figures are not determined from malpractice claims by patients—a crude method which obviously grossly underestimates the true number of complications, which is exactly the point here.

On page 102 of his book *Chiropractic Malpractice*, chiropractor Peter Modde lists some of the other potential complications of spinal manipulation: Permanent joint damage, spinal cord injury, paralysis, cardiac arrest, and death. In the medical journals there are more than eighty citations regarding injury from spinal manipulation, most of them having to do with stroke victims. On the subject of "neck manipulation as a cause of stroke," James T. Robertson, M.D., reported that a survey of the Stroke Council of the American Heart Association turned up 360 previously unreported cases of strokes from neck manipulation.

The Cervical Vertebrae and the Right Vertebral Artery

The vertebral arteries thread through holes in the six upper cervical vertebrae where they are particularly vulnerable to rupture by the shearing force of a shift of one of those vertebrae in relation to the others. An artery tear so near the brain may cause brain tissue death and the horrific effects of stroke.

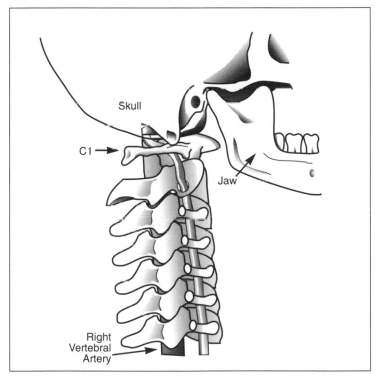

Drawing by Grafikus.

It should be emphasized that many of these tragedies were caused by treatment for such relatively minor problems as a stiff neck, or neck muscle pain, or, even more pathetic, by "preventive maintenance" adjustments where the victim was completely healthy and pain free. Some of them were caused by treatment which had no possible hope of relieving the problem at hand, such as neck manipulation for lower-back pain, or diabetes, or epilepsy, etc. Those are gratuitous injuries, being completely unnecessary and unjustifiable.

True Cases

Chiropractors are big on testimonials. Listen to these few:

Tina—"There had been no warning. Before I knew it I had blacked out. When I came to, I had double vision and I was *paralyzed*!! The chiro called a neurologist, but did not listen to the physician's advice. Instead of being taken to a hospital I was left in the office for over four hours. The chiro told me that I had only suffered a detached retina and that the paralysis was just a stress reaction. He still denies that I suffered a brain stem stroke, or that it was caused from having my neck manipulated."

George—"I went to a chiropractor for pain in my lower back. Amazingly, all his adjustments were on my neck, which was feeling fine—until after his seventh treatment. New pain suddenly developed in my neck and right shoulder, and there was continuous ringing in my ears. He couldn't fix it, so I went to three other chiropractors over the next few months. The third one not only couldn't correct the injuries, his adjustments left me with partial paralysis in my left foot, which has become painful to the touch. All of these injuries are permanent. Medical doctors cannot fix them either."

Sally—(Sally can't speak for herself; you see, she is dead. The attorney who handled her case will tell you what happened.)

Sally, "a 26-year-old housewife and new mother, entered a chiropractic office with her six-week-old daughter and requested treatment for a stiff neck that had been interfering with her breast-feeding and normal household activities. [The chiropractor] placed her in the supine, face-up position on his adjusting table, placed his hands on opposite sides of her head, and twisted her neck, first left and then right. Immediately following the adjustment, [Sally] complained to the chiropractor that she could not 'see straight' and was experiencing nausea and extreme headache. She was unable to raise her body from the table and the chiropractor immediately called an ambulance. She was hospitalized within four hours of the adjustment and died the next morning."

Victims of Chiropractic

Victims of Chiropractic doesn't want this suffering to be without purpose. VOC *purposes* are:

1. Mutual support. Experiencing injury from a licensed health professional is psychologically devastating, particularly if preceded by deceptive claims of effectiveness and safety.

2. Education of the public as to the health hazards of chiropractic.

3. Working to introduce and change state laws so as to require that prospective patients of chiropractors be informed about health risks, the realistic benefits, and viable alternatives.

Our *motivations* are:

1. The desire to bring some good purpose out of seemingly senseless tragedy.

2. The necessity to channel justified anger in a constructive way.

3. The desire to see evil (i.e., health care deception and irresponsibility) end.

4. The belief that the individual is important and worthy of being fully informed of the serious risks and the limited potential benefits of the unscientific practice of chiropractic, and that each person's health is valuable, worthy of respect and protection, and not properly an object of exploitation, nor to be considered dispensable.

5. Common decency gives the desire to not see anyone hurt (i.e., physical injury, diversion from appropriate medical treatment, or financial injury on worthless treatments).

Practical Suggestions

VOC believes that chiropractic is a significant hazard to many patients, and that significant reform of the profession is greatly warranted. Until such reform is instituted, what are our specific suggestions to you, the health consumers, in regard to chiropractic? These are our informed opinions:

1. "Since most back problems can be treated successfully without manipulation," [according to Robert L. Swezey and Annette M. Swezey], we recommend you try your family physician (an M.D.) first. He or she can refer you to a physical therapist (your best bet), or to an orthopedic physician, if your problem really is musculoskeletal. Other serious conditions not treatable or diagnosable by a chiropractor can cause back pain.

2. If they cannot help you, try to find a chiropractor who practices in harmony with scientific principles, rather than in contradiction of them, and limits his practice to the treatment of musculoskeletal problems. It is important to note that the credible studies favorable to chiropractic (i.e., Meade and RAND) have been strictly limited to *low-back* pain. Relief of musculoskeletal pain in other areas is plausible; relief of any other problems is not. If he (or his literature) claims that spinal manipulation can treat anything other than musculoskeletal problems of mechanical origin, if he spouts the disproven theory about subluxations impinging upon nerves or hindering energy flow, or if he has Parker-type nerve charts around, we strongly

suggest you go elsewhere. Such people are communicating to you that they believe in the conclusively false theory of their profession's spiritist founder, D. D. Palmer.

3. Do not submit to full-spine x-rays or to frequently repeated x-rays. They have been judged even by Andrew Weil, a physician sympathetic to some alternative health care, as "totally unnecessary," and they can cause cancer and genetic damage. "A routine set of spine x-rays in a young woman, for example, has a radiation effect on her ovaries equivalent to chest x-rays administered daily for sixty days," [according to Augustus A. White].

4. Do not accept nutritional advice or supplements from a chiropractor. Their advice has been judged by Victor Herbert, a renowned expert in the field, to be "exaggerate[d]" and "unscientific."

5. Do not submit to a long-term spinal adjusting schedule. "On the average after ten to twenty treatments, . . . the treatment itself can actually work as an irritant and perpetuate the original condition," [according to Peter J. Modde].

6. Be aware that neck manipulations are particularly dangerous. Make sure that the potential benefit justifies the risk of such manipulations.

Be Informed

In summary, be an informed, intelligent health consumer. Only by doing so can you minimize your chances of winding up as a statistic on some uncaring malpractice insurer's tote board of maimed lives. Without question the system is presently set up to tolerate deception and protect the chiropractors, not you. Many of the undiscerning have lived to regret their *trust* of a profession which often does not treat human health as very valuable.

Periodical Bibliography

The following articles have been selected to supplement the diverse views presented in this chapter.

Arline Brecher	"Can Vitamins Save Your Life?" *New Age Journal*, February 1993.
Vern L. Bullough and Bonnie Bullough	"Therapeutic Touch: Why Do Nurses Believe?" *Skeptical Inquirer*, Winter 1993.
Janet Bennett Clark	"Alternative Medicine Is Catching On," *Kiplinger's Personal Finance Magazine*, January 1993.
Henry Dreher	"Proven Mind/Body Medicine," *Natural Health*, May/June 1993.
Arielle Emmett	"Where East Does Not Meet West," *Technology Review*, November/December 1992.
William G. Flanagan	"Me and Dr. Gong," *Forbes*, December 9, 1991.
Valerie Frankel and Ellen Tien	"A Hard-Hitting Look at New Age Health," *Mademoiselle*, May 1992.
Adriane Fugh-Berman	"The Case for 'Natural' Medicine," *The Nation*, September 6-13, 1993.
Newsweek	"Healing and the Mind," special section, February 22, 1993.
Stephen Perrine	"The Crystal Healer Will See You Now," *Men's Health*, July/August 1993.
Anastasia Toufexis	"Dr. Jacobs' Alternative Mission," *Time*, March 1, 1993.
Anastasia Toufexis	"The New Scoop on Vitamins," *Time*, April 6, 1992.
Claudia Wallis	"Why New Age Medicine Is Catching On," *Time*, November 4, 1991.
Joseph Wassersug	"Keep Holistic 'Care' and Send a Surgeon," *American Medical News*, July 22, 1991. Available from 515 N. State St., Chicago, IL 60610.
Pat Wingert and Barbara Kantrowitz	"An Industry Unmonitored," *Newsweek*, June 7, 1993.

How Should the United States Reform its Health Care System?

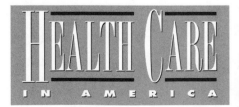

Chapter Preface

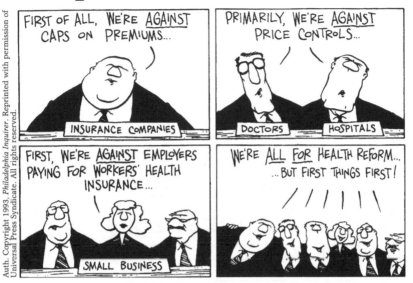

Patients, physicians, businesspeople, insurance representatives, and government workers are just a few of the people needed to run America's health care system. But as the cartoon above shows, these people often have conflicting interests and conflicting ideas about how to reform health care. These conflicts make reforming the system a complex, difficult challenge.

For example, many advocates support a single-payer approach to health care. The "single payer" would be the government, which would pay physicians, hospitals, and other health care providers directly. (Currently, many consumers pay for private health insurance and the insurance companies pay for patients' health care.) Physician Thomas Bodemheimer speaks for many single-payer supporters: "A single-payer model can provide equal health insurance for everyone at a reasonable cost."

Insurance companies oppose the single-payer plan for it would make them obsolete. But many other Americans also oppose a single payer. Most object to increased government involvement—they believe government-run plans are inefficient and costly and that the quality of care would decrease. As the Heritage Foundation's Peter J. Ferrara warns, "Unnecessary government regulation and control . . . would ultimately fail to . . . control costs."

Satisfying the demands of all Americans will not be an easy task. The following chapter presents a variety of proposed reforms designed to address the problems of America's health care system.

"Nationalization of the health care system would save both lives and money."

The United States Should Nationalize Health Care

Steffie Woolhandler and David U. Himmelstein

In many industrialized nations, the government pays for the health care of all its citizens. In the following viewpoint, Steffie Woolhandler and David U. Himmelstein argue that the United States should adopt such a system of nationalized medicine. The authors believe that nationalizing America's health care would eliminate the need for private insurance companies, thereby saving money. This savings could then be spent on improving the health care of all Americans. Woolhandler and Himmelstein are physicians who teach at the Harvard Medical School in Cambridge, Massachusetts.

As you read, consider the following questions:

1. Why do the authors believe a cost-effectiveness approach to health care reform would be wasteful?
2. Woolhandler and Himmelstein provide some examples of how nationalized health care systems have benefited the British and the Canadians. Cite two of these examples for each system.
3. How would the authors address the problem of expensive malpractice litigation?

From "Socialized Medicine Is Good Business," by Steffie Woolhandler and David U. Himmelstein, *In These Times*, January 25, 1993. This article originally appeared in the anthology *Why the United States Does Not Have a National Health Care Program*, edited by Vicente Navarro, M.D., and is reprinted with permission of Baywood Publishing Company, Amityville, New York.

In a report issued in January 1993, the Commerce Department said that spending on health care in 1992 reached a record 14 percent of the nation's total economic output, and predicted that by 1994 health care costs for the nation would total more than $1 trillion.

In simple human terms, uncontrolled increases in health care costs have caused millions of Americans to forgo needed health care or to be bankrupted as a result of health emergencies. For federal and state budgets, the increases mean less money available for investment in education, infrastructure and other needs. For business, especially small business, the burden of health insurance has become increasingly difficult to bear.

At his December 1992 economic town hall meeting in Little Rock, Arkansas, President Clinton said that bringing down health care costs was a prerequisite to other essential economic reforms. But in his campaign, Clinton also said that he wanted to rely on market forces as much as possible, and he praised managed competition among insurers as a strategy to control costs. Managed competition, however, would leave existing industry structures intact and could attain savings only by limiting the volume of clinical services or the wage cost of health workers. Managed competition is unlikely to provide adequate health care coverage for those now uninsured or underinsured, or to effectively control costs.

As long as health care remains a commodity, in which access to care is based on ability to pay, the inefficiencies and administrative waste of the current system will prevent substantial improvement in coverage or reduction in costs. Aside from being inherently unjust, differential access to health care based on ability to pay requires the herculean administrative task of attributing each charge and payment to an individual patient. This compels health institutions to waste huge amounts of money on marketing and bureaucratic sieves that separate lucrative from unprofitable patients, services and procedures.

Need-Based Care

The abolition of billing for service would with a single stroke eliminate the need for the entire insurance industry and much of doctors' office and hospitals' administrative expenses. Distribution of funds based on health care needs, rather than market forces, would save the money now spent on marketing. Eliminating corporate profit from the sale of health care would free up money for expanded health services and research. And abandoning litigation in favor of no-fault compensation for medical errors could direct remuneration to victims rather than attorneys and insurance companies.

In contrast to these reforms, most mainstream health policy

debate has concentrated on the optimal means of rationing care. Cost-effectiveness analysis is usually advocated as the way to minimize the ill effects of such rationing, but these analysts base their calculations on current costs, which include the sums wasted on bureaucracy, marketing, profits, high physicians' incomes and defensive medicine.

Based on the assumption that the health care system will remain essentially unchanged, the cost-effectiveness approach ignores the potential for saving through structural reform. Worse, the solution of rationing based on such analysis entails the collection of detailed financial data, additional administrative controls and further bureaucratic hypertrophy. In other words, additional administrative costs.

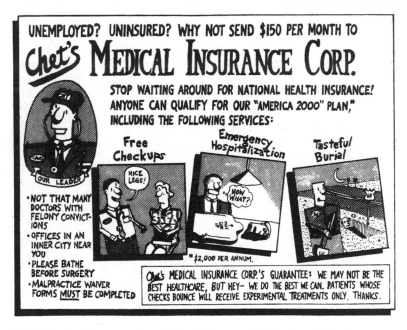

Ted Rall. Reprinted by permission of Chronicle Features, San Francisco, California.

The extent of waste in our current health care system is much greater than most people realize. Conservatively, we estimate that 30 percent of health spending ($226 billion in 1991) is wasted on administration, profits, high physician incomes, marketing and defensive medicine, none of which goes to improve health care.

Everyone now acknowledges that health care costs are higher

in the United States than in other industrialized nations. One of every seven dollars spent in the United States—14 percent of gross national product—goes to the health care industry. This compares to only 6 percent of gross national product for health care in Britain and 8 percent in Canada. And both those countries provide free care to all. Yet the advocates of managed competition claim that either a Canadian-style or a British-style universal health care system would be too expensive. Indeed, with the help of the media, they have created a popular perception that it would cost too much to provide uniform, free service to all Americans on the basis of need alone.

In fact, nationalization of the health care system would save both lives and money. A single-payer plan that eliminated the unnecessary costs outlined below would not only be less expensive than our present system, but would also save enough money to provide quality care for everyone. Left critics of U.S. health care, however, have focused on inequalities, arguing that universal free access would improve health care. Few have challenged the official ideology that the "free market" in health care engenders efficiency.

As a result, advocates of socialized medicine have not experienced the issue of skyrocketing costs as an opportunity, but as an obstacle. Yet the true obstacles to a national health service are not economic, but political and ideological. If the public understood the extent of waste in our current "free market" health care system, its days would be numbered.

High Costs, Poor Services

So let's look at the elements in the existing system that raise the cost of care without providing medical services.

First, administrative costs. Between 1970 and 1991, the number of health care administrators in the United States increased by 697 percent, while the total number of health care personnel increased by only 129 percent. Rapidly rising costs of health insurance overhead, hospital and nursing home administration and doctors' office overhead attest to the bureaucratization of medical care. In 1991 these costs totaled $159.1 billion, or 21 percent of all health care spending.

The 1,500 private U.S. health insurers took in $241.5 billion in premiums in 1991 and paid out $209.2 billion in benefits. The $32.3 billion in overhead paid for processing bills, marketing, building and furnishing insurance company offices, and profits for commercial insurers. In addition, the administrative costs of Medicare and other government programs totaled $10.3 billion.

Hospital administrative costs are more difficult to quantify because many personnel classified as clinical for accounting purposes do some administrative work. Internists in one academic department of medicine, for example, spend 18 percent of their time on administration, and social workers at many hospitals devote considerable effort to insurance reimbursement problems. But even excluding the administrative work of clinical personnel, vast amounts of money and human talent are expended on billing, marketing, cost accounting and institutional planning. In California, administration and accounting constitute 20.6 percent of hospital costs. Similar figures have been reported for hospitals in Florida and Texas. We estimate that, nationwide, hospital administration and accounting cost $57.6 billion in 1991.

In addition, nursing home administration accounted for 15.8 percent of total costs in California's long-term care facilities, and a similar proportion of Texas' nursing home costs. Using the California percentage projected onto the $59.1 billion spent nationally for nursing home care, we estimate administrative costs of $9.3 billion.

Finally, physicians incurred professional expenses of $66.8 billion in 1991, 45 percent of their gross income. Much of this is for administration. Secretarial and clerical staff make up 47 percent of non-physician personnel employed in doctors' offices. Much of their time is spent on tasks like patient and third-party billing.

These administrative costs have increased much more rapidly than overall health spending in recent years—16.4 percent compared to 10.3 percent for the most recent year for which we have figures. Costs of hospital administration have also risen much more rapidly than other hospital costs. At one major Northeastern teaching hospital, the proportion of total expenditures devoted to administration has doubled over the past 55 years. And so it goes across the board.

Simplified Billing

In contrast to all this, Canada's universal health insurance system, administered by the provincial governments, gives each hospital a single annual lump sum to cover operating expenses and pays doctors on a fee-for-service basis. Capital spending is tightly controlled, and binding fees are negotiated between the government and physicians. A Canadian hospital has virtually no billing department and little of the detailed internal accounting structure needed to attribute costs and charges to individual patients and physicians. Physician billing is simplified by the unified system, with overhead averaging only 0.9 percent of premium income, one-fourteenth of the U.S. private insurers' overhead.

In Canada, administration accounts for only 9 percent of hospital spending. Insurance overhead and hospital administration together consume 6 percent of total Canadian health resources.

In Britain, the National Health Service owns most hospitals, pays physicians on a salaried or capitation basis and has no insurance overhead. Administrative costs there amount to 5.7 percent of hospital expenses and central administration consumes 2.6 percent of total spending. Together these categories account for 6 percent of health spending, though recent market-oriented reforms may drive up these figures.

Most Americans Want Nationalized Health Care

Nearly every poll in the past 30 years has shown that a majority of Americans support a universal, comprehensive, publicly-administered health service of the kind that exists in Canada and western Europe.

In 1988, exit polls revealed that even a majority of Bush voters supported national health insurance.

In 1990, two-thirds of those polled said they would prefer a nationalized health-care system like Canada's and 73 percent favored an increase in public health spending.

Phil Gasper, *Socialist Worker*, April 1993

Comparing the Canadian and British systems to our own, we calculated the potential administrative savings in the U.S. would be $115.2 billion—15.2 percent of current health spending—using the Canadian system, and even more using the British system.

In addition to these potential administrative savings, separating corporate profit from health care could save substantial sums. Profits of health-related industries have soared in the past three decades. After-tax profits averaging 7.6 percent between 1978 and 1983 placed health care third among the 42 U.S. industry groups.

Profits represent health spending in excess of the costs of care, and there is no evidence to suggest that higher profits mean better care. Indeed, the scant empirical evidence comparing proprietary and not-for-profit hospitals and nursing homes supports the opposite conclusion.

Similarly, claims of greater efficiency in the for-profit health sector are not supported by current data. Private insurance plans have much higher overhead than do government insurance programs. For-profit hospitals economize on clinical personnel and services but have higher total per diem costs because of greater administrative and ancillary services.

Decreased Effectiveness

The pursuit of profit also diminishes the cost effectiveness of the health care system as a whole by basing resource allocation primarily on financial considerations. The profit-maximizing behavior of medical enterprises often conflicts with the cost-minimizing interests of society. Long-term cost-effective services that offer scant financial reward—immunization programs, prenatal care for the poor, nonpharmacologic treatment of borderline hypertension—remain underdeveloped. But vast resources are devoted to lucrative but unproven services such as executive stress tests, weight-loss clinics and coronary artery surgery.

Pharmacological firms also squander enormous sums promoting "me-too" formulations of popular drugs, while eschewing vaccines or "orphan" drugs for uncommon illnesses. Similarly, the option of home-based renal dialysis is unavailable in many areas, forcing all dialysis patients into institute-based treatment, which is twice as expensive (and more profitable).

Adopting the British model of nationalization or a Canadian-style tightly controlled public insurance system in the United States would largely eliminate the profits of health care providers ($2.8 billion in 1983) and financial institutions ($2.1 billion in 1983). Broader reform could curtail profits in drugs ($5.6 billion), medical equipment ($2.8 billion) and hospital construction ($200 million). Thus potential savings from eliminating health care profits range from $4.9 billion to $13.5 billion, depending on whether nationalization was limited to health providers or was extended to suppliers and construction as well.

Physicians' incomes make up another area of potential savings. In 1941, doctors in the U.S. earned 3.5 times as much as average workers. This ratio had climbed to 6.0 in 1990, when doctors' incomes averaged $164,300. We are unaware of any improvement in the quality of care as a result of this increase, and 70 percent of Americans now believe that doctors are overpaid. Further, current reimbursement mechanisms skew the distribution of physician services toward financial rather than health needs and have increased disparities between primary care providers and specialists.

The impact of a national health program on physician incomes would depend on the fee or salary scale. In 1982, the average Canadian doctor earned $97,000 (Canadian dollars), 4.8 times the average wage, and disparities among specialists were considerably smaller than in the United States. Inter-speciality inequalities are also smaller in Britain, where in 1980 the average physician earned 2.3 times the average male worker's wage. If U.S. doctors' incomes were reduced to the level found in Canada or England, savings of $20.4 or $44.9 billion would be achieved.

Saving Money on Drug Advertising

Drug marketing is yet another source of potential savings—to the tune of at least $4 billion now spent on advertising and "detailing." Some argue that such marketing is not only expensive, but that it also adversely affects physicians' prescribing habits. Similar arguments apply to advertising for medical equipment and supplies.

Advertising by hospitals, HMOs and other health providers has increased dramatically in recent years. Hospital industry sources estimate that advertising and marketing account for 1 percent of total not-for-profit spending and between 3 and 5 percent of for-profit spending. Based on these figures, provider marketing costs at least $3.4 billion in 1991. Total marketing and advertising costs exceeded $7.4 billion in 1991. If reimbursement under a national health program excluded compensation for such activity, at least that much more could be saved.

And finally, we have the legal profession, which has become increasingly entangled in health care. The legal complexity of medical practice and administration now requires many hospitals to retain full-time legal counsel. Malpractice litigation and so-called defensive medicine (excessive diagnostic testing) consume considerable physician time and expense, with malpractice premiums alone costing $5 billion in 1983.

The effect of malpractice litigation on the quality of care is at best uncertain. Litigation is an inefficient and capricious way to assure quality care. Between 66 and 80 percent of malpractice premiums are consumed by legal costs and insurance overhead, yet while 8 percent of doctors are sued each year, fewer than 300 verdicts favor the patients. Even assuming that many cases are settled without trial, the financial benefits to patients are tiny compared with those to lawyers.

A national no-fault compensation system for iatrogenic damage or error, modeled on the Swedish malpractice system or New Zealand's accident compensation system, would compensate patients more fairly and reduce legal fees. Considerable savings would also result from the abolition of incentives for defensive medicine, estimated to cost about $15 billion annually. Based on the lower figure, and assuming that some of this potential saving has already been included in our calculation of administrative costs and profits, legal reform might yield savings of at least $15 billion.

In the light of all of the above inefficiencies and waste—amounting to some $138 billion by our most conservative estimates—it is striking that most health care "experts" see cost control and equality in health care as contradictory. We believe that any honest comparison of our current system to those of the countries closest to us in culture and history clearly shows the superiority of socialized medicine. We think that most Americans would prefer such a system to the preservation of a private system that protects profit and privilege while remaining blind to waste and want.

"Socialized medicine takes away our control over our own health and body, and gives that power to the state. "

Nationalized Health Care Would Be Disastrous

Jarret B. Wollstein

Socialized, or nationalized, medicine is inefficient and expensive, contends Jarret B. Wollstein in the following viewpoint. Wollstein maintains that Britain, Canada, and other nations with nationalized medicine have poorer quality care than does the United States. The author concludes that Americans need *less* government intervention in health care, not more, if they are to establish a cost-effective system that meets everyone's health care needs. Wollstein is a director of the International Society for Individual Liberty, which advocates free-market economics, individual liberty, and other libertarian doctrines.

As you read, consider the following questions:

1. What specific problems have Britain and Canada had with socialized medicine, according to the author?
2. Why is America's health care system in crisis, in Wollstein's opinion?
3. What suggestions does the author have for reforming America's health care system?

From "National Health Insurance: A Medical Disaster" by Jarret B. Wollstein, *Freeman*, October 1992. Reprinted with permission.

Affordable health care has become one of the most important social issues of our time. Every news broadcast seems to have a special report on "America's health care crisis" or a politician demanding "universal health insurance." Evidence cited for the need for immediate and drastic government action includes:

High medical costs. The United States reportedly has the highest per capita medical expenditures of any country in the world. According to *Insight* magazine, U.S. citizens spent an average of $2,051 on health care in 1990, compared to $1,483 for Canadians and $1,093 for West Germans.

Rapid increase in medical expenditures. The average American now spends 11.1 percent of his income on medical care. If current trends continue, health care will consume over 17 percent of the Gross Domestic Product within 15 years.

High administrative costs. In the U.S., administrative costs consume nearly 12 percent of health dollars compared to 1 percent under Canada's socialized system. More than 1,100 different insurance forms are now in use in the United States.

Americans without insurance coverage. At any given time, over 13 percent of Americans have incomes that are too high to qualify for Medicare or Medicaid, but are too low to pay for medical insurance themselves.

The free market in health care, we are told, has failed. The solution offered by a growing chorus of commentators and candidates is *universal, mandatory, national health insurance;* in other words, *socialized medicine.* Is socialized medicine the answer, or will it only make things worse?

How Well Has Socialized Medicine Worked Elsewhere?

Most of the developed countries of the world presently have some form of socialized medicine. How well has it worked?

Great Britain. Great Britain adopted socialized medicine in 1948, with the creation of the National Health Service (NHS). The political rhetoric in Britain exhorting the adoption of nationalized health insurance is similar to what we are hearing in the U.S. today. In 1942, Prime Minister Winston Churchill declared:

> The discoveries of healing science must be the inheritance of all. . . . Disease must be attacked whether it occurs in the poorest or the richest man or woman, simply on the ground that it is the enemy. . . . Our policy is to create a national health service, in order to secure that everybody in the country, irrespective of means, age, sex, or occupation, shall have equal opportunities to benefit from the best and most up-to-date medical and allied services available.

With the adoption of national health insurance, Labour Minister Dr. David Owen predicted, "We were going to finance everything, cure the nation and then spending would drop." Unfortunately things didn't work out exactly as planned.

The first problem with Britain's National Health Service was skyrocketing demand. With health care paid for entirely by the government, there was no reason not to go to a doctor. Why take aspirin or wait out a cold, when professional medical care is free? As Michael Foot observed, within months "the demand [for health care] was exceeding anything [its creators] had dreamt of." First-year operating costs of NHS were 52 million pounds higher than original estimates.

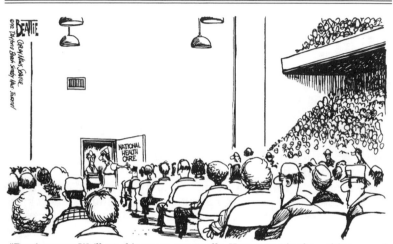

"Don't worry. We'll get this set up eventually. Have a seat in the waiting room."

Beattie/Copley News Service. Reprinted with permission.

NHS soon found itself in direct competition for funds with national defense, pensions, and all other governmental functions. Budget cuts for NHS quickly followed. British economists John and Sylvia Jewkes estimated that between 1950 and 1959 the United States spent six times more per capita on hospital construction than England. As a result, there was a steady deterioration in the quality of British medical care.

By 1977, British general practitioners rarely had any medical instruments except for stethoscopes and blood-pressure meters. They had to send their patients to hospitals even for such routine procedures as X-rays and blood tests. The waiting time for routine, non-emergency surgery had increased to years. By the mid-1970s, more than 700,000 English men, women, and children were on hospital waiting lists at any given time. The average British doctor now has over 3,000 patients, compared to 500-

600 for the average American doctor. NHS doctors spend an average of less than five minutes with their patients, who usually wait hours to see them.

In 1975 Bernard Dixon, then editor of the British magazine *New Scientist*, provided this summary of the state of National Health Insurance:

> The plight of Britain's Health Service conflicts desperately with the avowedly utopian ideals of its founders. For most of us, it is only when we join a year-long hospital waiting list, or have to take an injured child to a hospital casualty department, that we realize just how threadbare and starved financially the service really is. Not only is there an acute shortage of resources, but the expertise and facilities that are available are all too often dispensed via a conveyer-belt system which can at times be positively inhuman.

As a result of widespread public dissatisfaction, in 1989 the British government began dismantling its National Health Service, and reintroduced market-based health care competition.

Canada. What of the Canadian National Health System, which many U.S. politicians are now championing as a less expensive and more efficient alternative to our supposed free market system?

The Canadian Model

Canada has had socialized medicine for 20 years, and the same pattern of deteriorating facilities, overburdened doctors, and long hospital waiting lists is clear. A quarter of a million Canadians (out of a population of only 26 million) are on waiting lists for surgery. The average waiting period for elective surgery is four years. Women wait up to five months for Pap smears and eight months for mammograms. Since 1987, the entire country spent less money on hospital improvements than the city of Washington, D.C., which has a population of only 618,000. As a result, sophisticated diagnostic equipment is scarce in Canada and growing scarcer. There are more MRIs (magnetic resonance imagers) in Washington State, which has a population of 4.6 million, than in all of Canada, which has a population of 26 million.

In Canada, as in Britain under socialized medicine, patients are denied care, forced to cope with increasingly antiquated hospitals and equipment, and can die while waiting for treatment. Canada controls health care costs the same way Britain and Russia do: by denying modern treatment to the sick and letting the severely ill and old die.

Despite standards far below those of the United States, when variables such as America's higher crime and teenage pregnancy rates are factored out, and when concealed government overhead costs are factored in, Canada spends as high a percentage of its GNP [gross national product] on health care as the United States. Today a growing chorus of Canadians, including many former champions of socialized medicine, are calling for return to a market-based system.

The Worldwide Failure of Socialized Medicine

Throughout the world the story is the same: socialized medicine results in skyrocketing demand for nominally "free" health care, doctors are overburdened, medical services steadily deteriorate, and there are endless waiting lists for health care. In the Soviet Union before the collapse of Communism, anesthetics, painkillers, and most drugs were rationed; 57 percent of hospitals had no hot running water; and it was standard practice to clean needles with steel wool and reuse them. In New Zealand, which has a population of just 3 million, there is a waiting list of 50,000 for surgery.

Socialized medicine doesn't even fulfill its promise of equal access to treatment regardless of ability to pay. For example, in Canada "a small child with a skin rash is 22 times more likely to see a dermatologist if the child is living in Vancouver [a major city] than in the East Kootenay district [a remote rural area]." In Brazil, "residents of urban areas experience 9 times more medical visits, 15 times more related services, 2.7 times more dental visits and 4.5 times more hospitalizations," than do rural dwellers.

Throughout the world, there are more and more refugees from socialized medicine. Middle-class Canadians flock across the U.S. border to avoid waiting months or years for routine procedures. In England a system of private, quasi-legal clinics has developed to care for patients who can no longer tolerate the abysmal medical services provided by national health insurance. In Russia, desperate patients bribe doctors and secretly visit them after hours to get decent treatment and scarce drugs.

Socialized medicine, like all forms of socialism, has been a world-wide failure. As people throughout the world from the Soviet Union to South America are learning, socialism cannot work. Socialism is fundamentally incompatible with human nature.

Socialism fails because it denies and degrades our essential humanity by treating us as objects. Socialized medicine takes away our control over our own health and body, and gives that power to the state. Under a socialized medical system, the government, not you or your doctor, decides what treatments, doctors, and drugs you get. If you don't like the service the government gives you, your only alternative is to flee to another country or to break the law and bribe a doctor. Under socialized medicine, the exercise of free choice becomes a crime.

Even after it destroys quality health care and individual liberty, socialized medicine still cannot achieve equal treatment for all. When planners try to make all people equal, they confront the inescapable paradox of equality: Abolishing inequality requires massive government power. But power by its nature is unequal: there are those that have it and those that do not. Giving government the power to make everyone equal necessarily creates the worst form of inequality: that of master and subject. In practice under socialized medicine, those with more money and friends in the government get vastly better health care than those without power and connections.

Socialized medicine will not work any better in the United States than it has in England, Canada, Russia or elsewhere. Consider just the economics of socialized medicine in the U.S. Medicare and Medicaid costs are already skyrocketing out of control. State governments cannot afford the 20 percent of their budgets that Medicare and Medicaid now consume. Where will government get hundreds of billions of dollars more for national health insurance? A complete Canadian-style national health insurance system for the U.S. would initially cost over $339 billion and require that payroll taxes be nearly doubled, or require a new, national 10 percent business tax.

Socialized medicine does not work, but has the free market failed as well? If freedom works, why is American health care now in crisis?

Government Intervention and Health Care Costs

The answer is that America does not have a free market in health care, and in fact has not had one for 50 years. What we have had is a half century of mounting government encroachment upon medical freedom, leading to more and more health care problems.

Over 42 percent of funds spent on American medical care are now controlled by government. Over 700 state laws, some hundreds of pages long, govern all health care providers and institutions. According to some estimates, for every man-hour of health services provided by doctors, two hours are spent by clerks filling out government paperwork. Dr. Francis A. Davis estimated in the March 1991 issue of *Private Practice* that government regulations have already increased the cost of medical care by up to 50 percent!

Government regulations and controls now intrude upon virtually every area of health care in America. These regulations increase tremendously the cost of health care. . . .

Health Care Alternatives

Fortunately, socialism and inaction are not our only two options. We can make health care more affordable and more available while preserving quality and freedom of choice. Here are some positive steps we can take now:

Privatize Health Care. Medicare and Medicaid are imposing horrendous costs upon American taxpayers. There is no free lunch. When health care is "free" (i.e., indirectly financed by taxation), there is little incentive for either patients or doctors to minimize costs. Government-guaranteed medical services raise prices and costs, result in massive waste, and create a bureaucracy in a futile attempt to control costs.

Government should get out of the medical insurance business. We will get far better value for our health care dollars if we spend them directly ourselves.

Government Is a Poor Administrator

Government as an administrator in health care does not work. History has proven that. Let us not repeat the mistakes of the past. . . . Let government guarantee the right of all citizens to reasonable health care. Let government guarantee appropriate insurance for its citizens. Let government set the standards in reasonable care and public health needs. But let others administer the program outlined.

If we learn from history, we can create a system that will meet the demands of our people but not be doomed to ultimate failure by a lack of recognition of the pitfalls of government as an administrator.

Gary F. Krieger, *American Medical News*, October 5, 1992.

Free Insurance Companies from Government Regulations. Government insurance mandates—specifying how insurance policies must be written, what illnesses may be covered, and what fees can be charged—put a straitjacket on health insurance providers and cost the U.S. economy over $60 billion a year. There are now over 700 mandates enforced by state governments. These mandates prohibit inexpensive policies with limited coverage—leaving 8.5 million Americans uninsured.

Using medical insurance to pay for small claims is also highly inefficient. As Joseph Bast points out in *Why We Spend Too Much on Health Care*, "it costs as much as $50 to process a $50 claim," adding billions to medical costs.

Insurance companies should be free to innovate and introduce new policies which meet the diverse needs of the American people. Relieved of the governmental regulations currently imposed on them, health care insurers could become leaders in cutting costs and creating inexpensive coverage for currently uninsured

Americans. The single reform of ending all mandates would reduce health care insurance costs in the U.S. by 30 percent!

Deregulate Medical Research and Marketing. Burdensome government testing and certification requirements have added years of delay and billions of dollars in cost to the development and marketing of new drugs. Government has made it economically impossible for small pharmaceutical manufacturers to survive, or for any manufacturer to develop drugs for diseases that affect small population groups. Hundreds of thousands of lives have been needlessly lost as a result of delays and added costs imposed by government regulations. Drugs which could alleviate the suffering of millions are kept from the market because they don't meet the government's arbitrary standards.

The decision whether or not to take a drug should be made by the patient and his doctor. In a deregulated market, misleading or dangerous claims would be minimized by natural market forces, including the threat of legal action by consumers. Unlike government regulatory agencies which are protected from lawsuits for their mistakes by sovereign immunity, non-governmental businesses are always subject to legal action.

Deregulating medical research and marketing would save tens of thousands of lives a year, make it economical to develop many new drugs, and drastically cut the cost of drugs for everyone.

End Medical Monopolies. The American Medical Association is a coercive monopoly which makes it difficult or impossible for alternative health care providers—such as nurse-practitioners, midwives, osteopaths, chiropractors, and nutritionists—to market their services. State medical licensing boards are composed virtually entirely of AMA-certified physicians and have created "medical standards" which make it impossible for medical schools to survive unless they adopt curricula approved by the AMA.

AMA-dominated, politicized state medical licensing ought to be abolished and replaced by independent certification of doctors. Consumers, not politicians or powerful groups of doctors, should decide which health care practitioners we can patronize.

End Drug Prohibition. Drug prohibition is a contributing factor to America's health care crisis. Legalizing drugs would eliminate many deaths from adulterated substances, permit addicts to seek treatment without fear of arrest, enable those suffering from glaucoma and cancer to use marijuana and cocaine therapeutically, and permit patients and doctors to use drugs now legally available in other countries. Ending the war on drugs would reduce health care expenditures in the United States.

A Warning

If you want to know how national health insurance would work in America, we have a model. For more than 60 years the

Veterans Administration has been charged with handling the health needs of millions of disabled and discharged servicemen and women. With a fiscal 1990 budget of $30 billion, the VA runs America's largest health care system, including 172 hospitals, 233 outpatient clinics, and 122 nursing homes. Investigations of the VA have found abominable conditions: long waiting periods for surgery, filthy hospitals, severe shortages of staff and drugs, antiquated equipment, incompetent staff, indifferent and hostile administrators. Here is just one example:

On January 15, 1992, CBS News reported that Walter Reed Army/Navy Medical Hospital had been refusing to provide amputees coming back from the Gulf War with artificial limbs. Other veterans were given shoddy prosthetics using antiquated technology. Compounding the tragedy, Walter Reed refused to accept donations of modern prosthetics offered by sympathetic Americans.

Commenting on why soldiers were denied modern artificial limbs, a Medical Services colonel retorted, "I am not going to spend the taxpayers' money if you will just be sitting at home. Why should I spend $5,000 for something that you will just look on?" Commenting on the refusal of Walter Reed hospital to accept donations of modern limbs for veterans, the colonel stated, "We disapprove it because we are the primary health-care providers and we believe that we provide the best total care to the patient. And the patients belong to us."

The most callous Soviet bureaucrat could hardly have been more arrogant. This incident gives us a glimpse of the future of health care in America—if national health insurance is enacted.

"The Canadian model of health care [reminds us that we] can develop a system of health care for all."

The United States Should Adopt a System Similar to Canada's

Elaine Bernard

Elaine Bernard, past president of the New Democratic Party of British Columbia, Canada, is director of the Trade Union Program at Harvard University in Cambridge, Massachusetts. In the following viewpoint, Bernard defends Canada's health care system and argues that health care in the United States would dramatically improve if Americans followed Canada's lead. Canada's system, Bernard asserts, covers all Canadians and provides excellent benefits at a reasonable cost.

As you read, consider the following questions:

1. How is Canada's system controlled by both the national government and the provincial governments, according to Bernard?
2. What "common myths" about Canada's system does the author describe?
3. What specific lessons can Americans learn from Canada's experience with nationalized health care, in the author's opinion?

Excerpted from "The Politics of Canada's Health Care System: Lessons for the U.S." by Elaine Bernard, *New Politics*, Winter 1992. Copyright 1992, New Politics Associates, Brooklyn, New York. Reprinted with permission.

A widely used tactic in the current debate on health care reform in the U.S. has been to compare health care delivery in the U.S. with Canada's national health care system. For U.S. supporters of a national, universal, single payer health care system, the Canadian experience offers a working alternative which has been in operation for over 20 years. While Americans are generally loathe to look at foreign institutions as models for domestic reform, the close geographic proximity of Canada and the similarities in values, institutions and outlook between the two countries make Canada seem less foreign to Americans. Opponents of significant health care reform are quick to warn of the evils of socialized medicine, even in Canada, arguing that the adoption of such a system will mean long waiting lists for surgery, increased government interference in the relationship between patients and doctors, tax increases, and generally inferior medicine with less choice for patients.

With so much of the U.S. health care debate now pivoting on the "Canadian model," we think it is valuable to take a closer look at the origins of this system. We will look at the Canadian health care system with six questions in mind: why Canada? What exactly is the Canadian model? How was it achieved politically? What are some of the common myths about the Canadian model and what is the current status of the system? Finally, what can Americans learn from the Canadian model?

Why Canada?

Thirty years ago, there was no significant difference in the provision of health care in Canada and the U.S. Since 1971, however, the two countries have gone in dramatically different directions with dramatically different results.

To highlight some of the more important differences, in the U.S. over 37 million people are without health insurance and a further 53 million are underinsured, which means that they are inadequately insured in the event of a serious illness. Canada, by contrast, not only offers *all* of its residents comprehensive health care, but it does so at a far lower cost than in the U.S. While Canadians spend 8.7% of their Gross National Product on health care, or the equivalent of $1,483 (U.S.) per person, the U.S. spends 11.8% of the GNP, or $2,051 per person for a health care system that doesn't provide health care for all.

For Americans, health care coverage depends primarily on whether health insurance is provided by their employer or through two major public programs, Medicaid for the poor and Medicare for the elderly. For both public and private employees, health care benefits and cost vary tremendously. By making workers dependent upon their employer for health care, there is an extra burden on workers who are forced to change or lose their jobs in the U.S. Also, a growing number of people with a history of health problems, or with what insurance companies deem to be "pre-existing conditions," find themselves "uninsurable." With rising health care costs, many employers in the private sector do not provide any health care benefits at all. Most employers, whether private or public, are attempting to shift the cost of health care programs onto workers. Medicare now covers only about 40% of the health care costs of the aged.

All Canadians, rich and poor, regardless of the state of their health, age, or employment status, are covered by the same comprehensive system. Canadians go to the doctor of their choice and receive hospital care free. There are essentially no financial barriers to health care in Canada, and there is an ample supply of physicians. Private insurance that duplicates the comprehensive services covered by the provincial plans are prohibited. Co-payments, deductibles, and direct patient payments to providers for covered services are also not permitted.

What Is Canada's Health Care System?

The Canadian system is a carefully crafted hybrid reflecting the many political compromises entailed in adopting a major social program in face of a powerful opposition. The system can be described as a publicly funded, privately provided, universal, comprehensive, affordable, single-payer, provincially administered national health care system. To explain each of these components in turn, publicly-funded means that its operating revenues come out of government general revenues—taxes.

A provincially administered national program sounds contradictory, but in Canada, as in the U.S., there is a division of power between the federal and provincial levels of government, with health care designated a provincial responsibility. Federal legislation, the Canada Health Act, set out the basic guidelines for the system. The federal government encouraged provincial government cooperation by agreeing to pay 50% of the costs of provincially-administered systems which followed the national standards.

The health care system is administered in each province through a single public agency—the single payer—accountable to the provincial legislature. All provincial health care plans are required to be fully portable within Canada, which means there is reciprocal recognition of coverage between provinces. Universal access is defined to mean that no less than 95% of the eligible recipients in any province must be covered by the program.

Health care itself is privately provided, with the vast majority of doctors in private practice charging for care on a fee-for-service basis. Doctors' organizations annually negotiate the fee schedule with each provincial health care agency. The overwhelming majority of hospitals in Canada are private, non-profit. They receive global operating budgets from the provincial government. New capital expenditures are allocated separately.

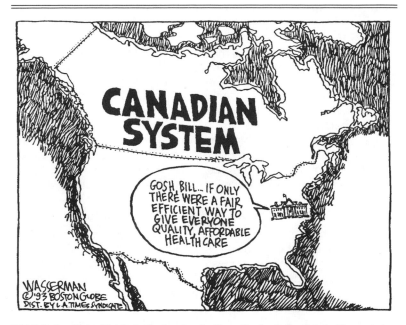

© 1993 Boston Globe. Distributed by Los Angeles Times Syndicate. Reprinted with permission.

To many Americans, the Canadian health care system could be a working model for an equivalent American system. In a recent national survey in the U.S., two-thirds of the respondents said that they would prefer the Canadian system to the one in the U.S. While identifying an appropriate model is useful, devising a political strategy to implement such a program is a far more challenging problem. Again, the Canadian example can provide some insight.

How Did They Get It?

The general principles of the national health care system were established in 1959 in the prairie province of Saskatchewan by Canada's social democratic party and predecessor to the New Democratic Party (NDP), the Cooperative Commonwealth Federation (CCF). Long committed to health care for all, the CCF was first elected as the provincial government in Saskatchewan in 1944. During its first term in office, in 1947, the CCF introduced a province-wide public hospital insurance plan. Within a few years, this program was sufficiently popular that the other provinces adopted similar schemes.

In 1958, the provincial and federal governments worked out an arrangement to share the costs of the provincial hospital insurance programs. In Saskatchewan, this meant that provincial funds were now freed up to undertake further health care reform. In the 1960 provincial election, the CCF/NDP promised to introduce a comprehensive provincial health care system. Voters were told that a system of comprehensive medical service coverage for all, with affordable premiums subsidized by general revenues, was now possible. This system would emphasize prevention and early diagnosis and treatment, and was to be coordinated with other existing health programs, such as hospital insurance. It was to promote medical research and education and to emphasize the value of human life. Finally, reflecting the concerns of a rural province, the program was to seek ways of encouraging the best distribution of doctors throughout the province.

The Doctors' Strike

The CCF won the 1960 election, in spite of a well-funded campaign by doctors in opposition to the health program. As the government proceeded to put its program into legislation through the Saskatchewan Medical Care Insurance Act (1961), the doctors continued their campaign against what they termed "socialized medicine." Accusing the government of "communism" and "compulsory state medicine," the doctors warned that the province was interfering with their right as professionals to practice medicine and was attempting to make them "salaried government employees." They warned that doctors would leave the province rather than work under such a system. Finally, in a last-ditch effort to force the government to back down on its health care reform, the doctors went on strike on July 1, 1961, the first day the new legislation came into effect.

The doctors' strike in Saskatchewan lasted 23 days and gained worldwide attention. While the doctors agreed to maintain emergency services and the provincial hospitals remained open with reduced staff, most private practitioners closed their offices. Ironically, the mortality rate in the province declined during the strike, primarily because of the decline in surgery.

While much of the national and international media condemned the doctors' action, the local media supported the doctors and demanded that the government back down on its program. In spite of the local media's support, as the strike wore on public opinion in Saskatchewan turned against the doctors. As communities started to recruit doctors willing to work under the health plan from other parts of Canada, the local doctors' resolve rapidly dwindled. The strike ended with the new health program still intact. The provincial government negotiated a face-saving agreement with the doctors which permitted them to opt entirely out of the plan and bill patients privately. With over 900 doctors in the province at the time, none chose this option. The agreement also permitted doctors to maintain their own medical insurance companies as clearinghouses for the Medical Care Commission, though these were eventually eliminated by the doctors themselves as needless duplication.

In spite of the controversial start to the Saskatchewan program, it quickly proved to be a success. Within a few years, the Saskatchewan model became the prototype for other provinces. Similar to what had happened with the groundbreaking initiative on hospital insurance, once the Saskatchewan model was in place the federal government passed legislation in 1966 which established the guidelines for a national health care system. The speed of the spread of the new system is impressive. By 1971, less than ten years after the introduction of the Saskatchewan system, every province in Canada had established a single-payer, universal, comprehensive health care plan.

Common Myths About the Canadian System

Adopting a system similar to the Canadian one means challenging powerful groups in U.S. society, specifically the insurance companies and the doctors. Both groups have lobbied politicians and commissioned studies to try to show that a U.S. national health insurance scheme modeled on the Canadian system would not work. They seek to convince Americans that they will get inferior health care coverage and fewer choices with a Canadian-type system.

An old charge, which is rapidly declining in its effectiveness but which is still sometimes heard, is that the Canadian system is "socialized medicine." The doctors in Saskatchewan made this charge at the time of its introduction. However, under a system of socialized medicine, doctors are salaried public employees rather than private practitioners. This clearly is not the case with the Canadian system, where 95% of the doctors are private and bill on a fee-for-service basis.

It may be worth noting, however, that from a socialist perspective, this is a problem with the Canadian system. While there is greater cost containment through the provincial health care agency negotiating the fee schedule, doctors in Canada—as in the U.S.—are still the gatekeepers in the system. And the fee-for-service system in both countries rewards doctors who perform more procedures and encourages doctors to perform unnecessary services to drive up their income.

Doctors in Canada have fared quite well under the national program. One important difference, though, which has led to considerable cost savings, is that while 75% of U.S. doctors are specialists, in Canada only 50% are specialists and the remainder are general practitioners. In both countries specialists charge significantly more than general practitioners and have higher earnings. Nevertheless, in Canada, in the five years preceding the introduction of the national health care system, physicians' incomes averaged 33.94% above the average for other professionals. For the five years following, their incomes surged to 47.02% above other professionals. Doctors still remain the highest paid professionals in Canada today. The fear that a national health care program may mean further "big government," administrative "red tape" and bureaucratic interference in the doctor/patient relationship is probably the most legitimate concern over "socialized medicine." Existing government-run health care programs in the U.S., which many people find inhibitingly complex, are hardly appealing models for a national system. One recent study revealed that 1 million Medicare enrollees a year find the claim process so complicated or time consuming that they do not seek reimbursement, losing about $100 million in benefits to which they are entitled.

Canada's System Works

Canada provides an attractive model for American reform. Canada (like most industrial democracies) combines universal health insurance with clear political accountability for raising and spending money for health services, and for the quality of the care the money buys. . . .

Primary and emergency care, universally insured, are readily available. No financial or administrative barriers prevent patients from seeking the services of any family doctor. Canadians are not assigned doctors from approved lists, but rather choose them. It is that simple.

Canadians visit physicians more often than Americans do and are highly satisfied with the service and the system. With a single insurer, the provincial government, there is far less paperwork for patients and doctors. More important is the widespread sense of security that comes from knowing that illness, however catastrophic, never results in financial disaster.

Theodore R. Marmor and John Godfrey, *The New York Times*, July 23, 1992.

On the charge of "big government," one of the major advantages of the Canadian single-payer system is its administrative efficiency and savings. Less than 3% of the expenditures in the Canadian system go to administrative costs. In the U.S., administrative costs consume over 15% of health care costs. The "free market" in health care in the U.S., with over 1,500 insurance providers with different fee schedules, wide variations in eligibility, co-payments, and deductibles, is an expensive and wasteful administrative maze, especially when compared to the simple, efficient Canadian system. Also, recent cost containment measures in American health care programs, such as "managed care," "preferred provider organizations" and "health maintenance organizations," have increasingly encroached upon patients' choices of doctors, treatment and services. Ironically, there is more choice in the Canadian publicly-run system, where patients may go to the physician of their choice and the physician need not worry about the patient's ability to pay for treatment.

Quality of Care

But what about quality of care? In Canada, we are warned, there is a lack of new technology and long waiting lists for care. Yet according to a 1991 report by the General Accounting Office of Congress on Canada's health insurance, "patients with immediate or life-threatening needs rarely wait for services, but waiting lists for elective surgery and diagnostic procedures may be several months long." Every country, including even the U.S., rations health care to some degree. The real issue is on what basis should this be done: ability to pay, or severity of need? Most Canadians who are sick or injured are cared for in a timely manner. Overall, rates of hospital use per capita are considerably higher in Canada than in the U.S. There are waiting lists for a few specialized operations in major Canadian cities. This is similar to the U.S., where some surgeons have long waiting lists for "elective" operations.

While Canada has a full range of high technology facilities, they are not as abundant as in the U.S. Access to expensive, high-technology medical equipment, such as magnetic resonance imaging and lithotripters (which generate shock waves to crush kidney stones) is more limited in Canada. This is because the provincial governments seek to control rising health costs by allocating the use of technology among hospitals in any given region. In the U.S., such decisions about the purchase of new technology are made by individual hospitals seeking a competitive advantage in the marketplace. This often leads to a proliferation of high-cost technology which is, arguably, unnecessary.

Measuring the overall quality of a service is somewhat difficult. One rather crude method used is to look at long-term indicators, such as death from heart disease, life expectancy, and infant mortality. Here again, Canada fares better than the U.S. Infant mortality deaths per 1,000 live births is 10.4 in the U.S., compared to 7.9 in Canada. Deaths from heart disease per 100,000 is

434 in the U.S. compared to 348 in Canada. Overall life expectancy in years is 75.3 in the U.S. and 77.1 in Canada. . . .

The single most important component of the Canadian system is its universality. Canadian progressives have attempted to build universality into all social programs because politically it is a unifying strategy. In the U.S., social programs tend to be targeted to specific groups and end up causing resentment among working people who feel that they must pay for these programs but cannot receive any benefits from them. This explains at least part of the "tax revolt" phenomenon in the U.S. Also, the target group receiving the benefit is usually relatively powerless and not able to mount a campaign to maintain the quality of the service they are receiving.

Universal programs are better able to assure quality for all by extending the service to socially powerful groupings. The poor and disadvantaged are included in the system with no social stigma of "special programs" attached to their rightful entitlement. Working people pay for the service with their taxes, but they also garner the benefits personally and directly. Canadians are adamantly opposed to a two-tier system, with a private system paralleling the public one, because it would allow the wealthy and powerful to buy superior care and reduce the pressure to maintain quality for all. Universality is a useful political strategy that builds social solidarity.

There has been much debate in the U.S. as to whether the states or the federal government should take the lead in initiating health care reform. The Canadian experience shows that while ultimately a national system is needed, a single state could lead the way with an exemplary model. In Canada, the CCF/NDP model in Saskatchewan set out the principles for the national system.

The Canadian experience also shows how quickly things can move once things get started. In less than 10 years after the introduction of the Saskatchewan system, Canada had a national health care program. One suspects that Americans will be equally anxious to universally adopt a comprehensive system once one state takes the initiative. . . .

Models such as the Canadian model of national health care are useful because they show us concretely that change is possible, and that there are alternatives to the current system which fewer and fewer Americans can afford. They remind us that we need not be victims of "the way things are" but, in fact, can develop a system of health care for all.

"If Americans are to achieve an affordable, universal, high quality health system, they cannot follow the Canadian path."

The United States Should Not Adopt a System Similar to Canada's

Edmund F. Haislmaier

Canada's health care system is plagued by rising costs and poor quality care, Edmund F. Haislmaier contends in the following viewpoint. Duplicating such a system in the United States, he believes, would only deepen America's health care crisis. Haislmaier is a policy analyst for the Heritage Foundation, a conservative think tank in Washington, D.C.

As you read, consider the following questions:

1. Haislmaier cites some examples of poor-quality health care in Canada. List a few of these examples.
2. What does the author mean when he states that Canada's health care system is separating into "two tiers"?
3. What type of health care system does Haislmaier advocate?

From "Problems in Paradise: Canadians Complain About Their Health Care System" by Edmund F. Haislmaier, The Heritage Foundation *Backgrounder*, February 19, 1992. Reprinted with permission.

Health care costs are escalating out of control. Families are finding it harder to obtain needed medical care. Spending on health care is taking a huge and growing bite out of federal and local government budgets, and the recession has made those budgets tighter. The spread of AIDS, the need for better treatment of drug and alcohol addiction, a chronic shortage of doctors in rural areas, and an aging population are imposing further burdens on the nation's health system.

Calls for health care reform thus are growing. Faced with demands for more government spending on health care, but with limited or declining funds to meet those demands, a number of government commissions are busy studying the mounting health care problems. Both in and out of government, critics complain there is too much waste in the system. They say it is too bureaucratic; that doctors make too much money; that they perform too many unnecessary tests and procedures.

A snapshot of America's health care crisis? No, it is a description of the health care debate in Canada—the very same Canada to which some American lawmakers look for a solution to America's health care problems. Just when some voices on Capitol Hill urge the United States to import Canada's universal, government-run health system, that system itself is sinking deeper into trouble and debt amid Canadian finger pointing and recriminations.

Eerie Similarity

To be sure, the Canadian health system has not yet reached the degree of crisis as in the U.S. But that day may not be far off. And while there are major differences between the U.S. and Canadian systems, there is an eerie similarity in some of the problems on both sides of the border. This similarity should induce more sober reflection by U.S. policy makers, particularly those inclined to advocate the adoption of a health system resembling Canada's.

In present day Canada unlimited demand for "free," government-funded medical care has collided headlong with limited public resources. As such:

• Canada's health system is plagued by soaring costs, with spending in recent years escalating at rates as great or greater than those of the U.S. system.

• The Canadian federal government, burdened with large budget deficits, is steadily reducing its share of funding for provincial health plans.

• Provincial health ministers are struggling to control their hemorrhaging budgets by closing hospital beds, laying off health workers, capping doctors' incomes, and limiting entry to medical schools.

• Provincial governments, including those headed by socialists, are trying to shift more health care costs to consumers by reducing or eliminating coverage for optional benefits and imposing user fees. Quebec's government is even considering adding to the taxable incomes of its citizens the value of the medical services they consume each year.

• Waiting lists are now endemic in Canada's health system, and a recent study estimates 260,000 Canadians are currently waiting for major surgery.

• In British Columbia, one of two provinces that charge citizens a monthly premium to help finance its health plan, between 2 percent and 5 percent of the population do not pay their premiums and thus technically are uninsured. These uninsured must pay doctors out of pocket for treatment or rely on charity care from physicians.

• When Robert Bourassa, the Premier of Quebec, needed cancer treatment, he crossed into the U.S. and obtained it at his own expense. Such actions by more affluent or politically well-connected Canadians raise the question of whether a "two-tiered" health system, of the kind Canadians long sought to avoid, is now emerging.

As Canadians increasingly debate the future of their health system and wonder how long it can survive in its present structure, the lesson for America should be clear. The existence of an ideal health system that offers unlimited, "free" government-funded medical care, while simultaneously limiting health spending without restricting patient choice or provider decision making, is a myth. If it ever did exist in Canada, it does not anymore. Pursuing the ephemeral mirage of a government-run health care Utopia never will lead to a high quality, low cost health system in America or anywhere else.

The Canadian Health System

Known colloquially as "medicare," Canada's universal, government-funded health system actually is a collection of similar systems operated by the provinces. Each of Canada's ten provinces and two territories administers its own universal health plan and pays for most of its costs. The main role of the Canadian federal government is to provide partial financing of the provincial health systems and to establish broad structural guidelines to which the provincial plans must adhere if they are to receive federal financial support.

Canadians take great pride in the fact that their health system gives all citizens access to care from hospitals and physicians that is free of charge to the patient at the point of service. While Canadians pay high taxes to fund this system, it is a price which, at least until now, the vast majority of Canadians have been willing to pay. Since their country, moreover, is increasingly questioning its very existence as a single nation, many

Canadians view their medicare system as a unifying institution. And many Canadians are proud that, at least in health care, their nation of 26 million is widely regarded as superior to its overbearing southern neighbor.

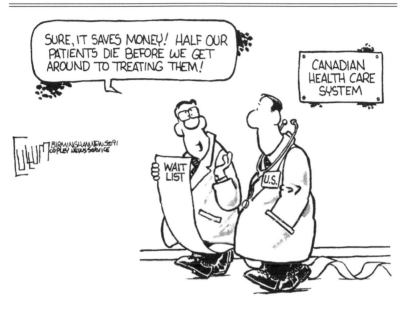

Cullum/Copley News Service. Reprinted with permission.

A growing number of Americans, including many members of Congress, look with envy at Canada's health system. Conscious of the 35 million Americans who lack health insurance, and the U.S. health system's dubious status as the world's most expensive, they see in their neighbor to the north a health system that provides universal coverage at a lower cost.

But all is not well in what some Americans view as Canada's health care paradise. While it is still all but unheard of for a Canadian to call publicly for scrapping or privatizing medicare, complaints are becoming louder and proposed reforms more sweeping in their scope. The major cause for Canada's growing health care debate: Soaring health care costs. . . .

No Reason for American Envy

Indeed, if misery loves company, then Americans and Canadians can find in each other good company when it comes to skyrocketing health care costs. While it is still commonplace to argue on both sides of the border that, in comparison with

America, Canada's health system delivers more care for less money, that comparison is increasingly misleading.

It is, of course, true that Canada gives almost all its citizens health insurance coverage, while an estimated 35 million Americans are uninsured for at least some period in any year. It is also true that Canada spends less than the U.S. on health care, as measured in per capita terms or as a percentage of each country's respective gross domestic product (GDP)—even though that difference has been greatly exaggerated.

But broader comparisons show that the margin of difference in health spending between the U.S. and Canada offers little reason for American envy or Canadian pride. The simple fact is: America may have the most expensive health system in the world, but Canada has the world's second most expensive system.

While most Americans are ignorant of this budget fact, more and more Canadian taxpayers are grimly aware of it. Explains Dr. Martin Barkin, former deputy health minister for Ontario, who argues that the current woes of Canadian health care cannot be blamed on underfunding:

> Canada is now the highest per-capita spender on health care of any country with a national health system. Amongst industrialized nations, only the United States, which doesn't have a government-run system covering all citizens, spends more—with worse results.

Similarly, Diane Francis, a columnist for *Maclean's*, Canada's leading news magazine, states flatly, "Proponents of Canada's medical myth should contemplate the fact that our costs are growing exponentially and are now the second-highest per capita in the world, after the United States."

When health care spending trends are analyzed, the future of the Canadian health system is as bleak as that of its U.S. counterpart. In both countries, the rates of growth in health care costs are outstripping general inflation rates by wide margins. Indeed, comparative data show that, during the 1970s and 1980s, the rates of growth in real (inflation adjusted) per capita health spending in the two countries have been virtually identical. In fact, real per capita health spending has grown faster in Canada than in the U.S. in recent years.

The lesson for America should be clear. Genuine success in bringing soaring health care costs under control will require a far better solution than simply adopting a national health system modeled on Canada's experience. . . .

Access to What and for Whom?

While all Canadians have access to government health insurance, the growing question is how much access to medical care—and of what kind—does that health insurance provide.

The *Wall Street Journal* in December 1991 reported that at Montreal's Royal Victoria Hospital tight budgets mean that the wait for a cataract/lens replacement is about three months, and for a coronary bypass it is between three and six months. In addition:

Tight budgets put extra strain on patients and staff. The hospital saves $660,000 a year by using an older type of injectable dye for X-rays that is less comfortable for patients than a newer dye. It bought new beds with manual cranks instead of electric motors. That means that the Royal Vic's 1,000 nurses must work a little harder every time they have to raise or lower a bed and patients can't just push a button to do it for themselves. On the maternity floor, it is strictly BYOD—bring your own diapers. The hospital stopped handing out free ones eight years ago.

A weekend here [in the emergency room] shows what happens when all the problems of Canadian health care converge. The ophthalmoscope and otoscope next to each bed that doctors use to examine patients' eyes and ears don't always work. Sometimes it takes hours to get a specialist to come down from a ward for a consultation, complains Francois Giumond, an emergency room doctor.

According to *The Christian Science Monitor*, in November 1991 at Toronto's Sunnybrook Health Science Centre:

A heart-disease patient categorized as an emergency case gets an operation within 48 hours. The wait lasts up to a week for urgent patients, up to six weeks for semi-urgent patients, and up to four months for elective patients.

Hospital officials are quick to point out that the system does accommodate patients who suddenly become emergency cases. In a few cases, though, the delay has proved fatal. To avoid the wait, some Canadians cross the border and have the operation in a U.S. hospital, where no such waiting lines exist. . . .

Most of the evidence of declining access and long waiting lists is anecdotal. However, preliminary findings of a privately sponsored survey of waiting lists in five provinces in 1991 revealed that an estimated 260,000 Canadians were waiting for major surgery. The equivalent in the U.S. would be 2.4 million Americans waiting for major surgery.

What should perhaps be most disturbing to Canadians is evidence that their health system is separating into "two tiers." The widespread and strongly felt desire to avoid a two-tiered health system was the principal reason why Canadians turned to universal government financing of health care in the first place. This now seems to be changing. Thus when Quebec Premier Robert Bourassa in August 1990 learned that he needed an operation for melanoma, a potentially fatal skin cancer, he chartered a plane at his own expense and flew to Washington, D.C., for a consultation at the National Cancer Institute in Bethesda, Maryland. In November, he returned to Bethesda for the operation, which was a success. Such treatment options are not generally available to less wealthy or politically well-connected Canadians—or for that matter, to Americans.

Uninsured Canadians

What might come as the biggest surprise to Americans is the existence of uninsured Canadian citizens. In the two provinces that charge health care premiums, Alberta and British Columbia, citizens who fail to pay technically are uninsured. While Alberta actually reimburses hospitals and doctors anyway for treating uninsured patients, as do many U.S. states, in British Columbia only the hospitals get reimbursed. This is because, as in all Canadian provinces, the government gives each hospital a fixed, annual (or "global"), budget, regardless of whom it treats. But the uninsured must pay for physician care out-of-pocket, or the doctors treating them must absorb the loss.

A Failed System

Canada's health system is lumbering toward disintegration and is posed to self-destruct. . . . Dr. Robert Macmillan, head of health insurance for the Ontario Ministry of Health, was quoted in *Forbes* as saying: "All of Canada faces a lag in accessibility, particularly in highly sophisticated care."

Perhaps the most visible result of Canada's single-payer system has been the forced rationing of health care. . . .

In addition to availability of care, costs have escalated to $8,600 per year for a family of four, and have added substantially to Canada's staggering national debt: on a per capita basis, Canada's total combined federal and provincial budget deficit is nearly double that of the U.S.'s combined federal and state deficit. . . .

Single-payer national health insurance based on the Canadian model would be a major disaster for the U.S.

Jerome C. Arnett Jr., *The Wall Street Journal*, August 6, 1993.

Various estimates put the uninsured population of British Columbia at between 2 percent and 5 percent, or 50,000 to 100,000 individuals. Were this figure applied to all of Canada, some 530,000 to 1.3 million people would be uninsured. And were this figure then transposed to the U.S., some 5 million to 12.5 million Americans would be uninsured—this is still a significant one-sixth to one-third of the present U.S. uninsured population. The British Columbia Medical Association estimates that each year its member doctors provide $15 million to $50 million in uncompensated care to the uninsured.

Canada at the Crossroads

The picture emerging from Canada is of a health system at the crossroads. Escalating costs and deteriorating access soon may force Canada to make a fundamental choice about the future of its health system.

One option is to introduce market-based reforms. The likely path would be a series of gradual steps such as the imposition of user fees and premiums, removal of restrictions on doctors and hospitals billing patients directly for all or part of their treatment, and the reintroduction of private insurance. Eventually, the government program could be means-tested—serving only the poor—with possibly some tax relief for private care and insurance purchased by the middle class.

Robert Evans, a Canadian health economist, points out that such a development essentially would mean the end of Canada's national health insurance experiment, and a return to where Canada was thirty years ago. This, says Evans, is where "the Americans have been all the way through."

The other scenario is to introduce ever tighter controls, restrictions, and rationing throughout the system, making doctors salaried employees of the government and drastically limiting Canadians' freedom of choice in medical care. Such a scenario would mean that Canada effectively would nationalize not only the financing of health care, but its delivery as well. The resulting system would resemble the heavily bureaucratic, centralized, and unresponsive national health systems found in Britain and Sweden. . . .

Lessons for America

The lessons for America in Canada's health care crisis should be clear. Ultimately, a government-run health system does not hold the hope of both restraining health care costs and expanding access to health care. While such systems may provide universal access to health insurance, and may initially bring some savings, inevitably, over time they prove that they can only control costs by denying access to medical care.

In the final analysis, access to health insurance is meaningless if it does not also give access to medical care. Contrary to the fond hopes of many Americans, including some members of Congress, Canada's national health system is finding that it is no exception to this rule.

If Americans are to achieve an affordable, universal, high quality health system, they cannot follow the Canadian path. The way to genuine reform of America's health system lies in consumer choice and true market competition, coupled with more effective government assistance for the needy and disadvantaged.

In theory, every health system in the world exists to serve patients and consumers. But the only way to make that theory a reality is by giving consumers direct control over the finances of the system. Only when individual consumers pay the piper will health care providers and health insurers dance to the tune of consumer demand. And only then will the providers and insurers offer the combination of low prices and high quality every health care consumer desires. It turns out that the Canadian health care paradise of unlimited, high quality, "free" government-funded medical care, combined with limited, controlled health care spending, is a mirage. Such a system does not and cannot exist.

"I recommend . . . 'managed competition.' Its purpose is to reward . . . health plans that provide high-quality care and effectively control cost."

Managed Competition Would Improve America's Health Care System

Alain C. Enthoven

In the debate over health care reform, many experts have advo cated a system of managed competition, in which large health maintenance organizations (HMOs) would compete to provide health care to individuals and businesses. In the following view-point, Alain C. Enthoven promotes managed competition as the best way for Americans to get high-quality, cost-effective health care. Enthoven, a professor at Stanford University in California, has written widely on economics, health care, and systems analysis, and is considered one of the architects of managed competition.

As you read, consider the following questions:

1. Why is fee-for-service an inefficient way to pay physicians, according to Enthoven?
2. What are "accountable health partnerships," as defined by the author?
3. Why does Enthoven oppose government-run health care?

"A Cure for Health Costs" by Alain C. Enthoven, *World Monitor*, April 1992. Reprinted with the author's permission.

American health care costs too much: more than $800 billion in 1992, approaching 14% of GNP [gross national product]. Canada and Germany get their health care for less than 9% of GNP, Japan and Britain for much less. In 1993 Americans will spend more than three times on health care what they'll spend on national defense, more than twice what they'll spend on education. These costs are straining public finances. *How and why has this happened?*

Medicare outlays for older Americans, about $88 billion in 1988, reached $130 billion in 1992. Medicaid outlays for poor people, $54 billion in 1988, were more than $104 billion.

Medical costs are a disaster for much of the US private sector. One of General Motors' big problems is an unfunded liability of $16 billion to $24 billion for retiree health care. The total for the whole private sector is well over $300 billion. These are resources that won't go into plant modernization or product engineering. America has too many hospital beds (they're about 64% occupied), too many medical specialists doing too much surgery, and too much high-tech equipment.

The US medical care system was not organized for quality and economy. It was organized to meet the conflicting professional and financial interests of doctors, hospitals, and insurance companies—and made worse by the inflationary way in which employers and unions buy medical care. There is practically no accountability for quality of care or costs, little incentive to do things in less costly ways.

Let me explain by contrasting the health-care system that we in America now *have* with the health-care system we *need*. I'll follow with some suggestions as to how we can get from here to there.

Adversaries with an 800 Number

The system we need would be made up of cohesive organizations attracting the loyalty, commitment, and responsible participation of doctors who would understand and accept the proposition that economy in health care is a worthy goal.

The system we have is an adversarial relationship between independent doctors and third-party payers. Most doctors feel no responsibility to control the costs to the third-party payer. They are taught that their first and only responsibility is to the patient.

An article in the *Journal of the American Medical Association* in 1989 reported that a majority of doctors would deceive the insurance company to get a claim paid if they felt it should be paid. Do a rhinoplasty (the cosmetic procedure known as a "nose job," usually not covered by insurance) but report it as a septoplasty (the presumably medically necessary procedure to open nasal air passages).

170

Doctors feel that restraints by third-party payers are an unwarranted infringement on their professional autonomy. Think how you would feel if you had decided your patient needed to be hospitalized, but first you had to call an 800 number and get permission from a computer-assisted nurse? The payers can't beat the doctors in such games. It's time to cut a different kind of deal.

Fee-for-Service or Fee-for-Efficiency?

The system we need would align the incentives of doctors and the interests of patients in high-quality economical care. Providers of medical care—doctors and hospitals—and payers would contract selectively for global units of care; that is, units based on person years (individual contract duration) or complete cases (operations, for example). The parties would agree on prices set in advance, with providers at risk for resource use; that is, taking the risk of any loss owing to their use or overuse of medical resources.

The Benefits of Managed Competition

Managed competition is one of several proposed strategies for fundamentally reforming health care. It emphasizes motivating consumers, insurers, and providers to be more cost-conscious, and it tries to imbue the health care system with the efficiency, flexibility, and innovation of competitive markets, without the undesirable outcomes of the present system. Much decisionmaking would remain decentralized. Managed competition would also pursue expanded or universal access to health insurance coverage. . . .

Managed competition would encourage consumers to be more price-conscious when making decisions about their health insurance. In turn, that would give insurers, and through them providers, motives to become more cost-conscious and efficient.

Congressional Budget Office, *Managed Competition and Its Potential to Reduce Health Spending*, 1993.

The Texas Heart Institute has made this approach famous: open-heart operations on a complete-case basis for a fixed price.

The system we have, based largely on fee-for-service payment, often pays more to poor performers than to good ones. Doctor A makes the correct diagnosis promptly and does the appropriate (i.e., best for the patient) procedure with skill and proficiency so the patient's problem is solved with no complications. Doctor B needs many repeated tests and visits to reach a diagnosis, does a procedure with poor proficiency, creates complications (like infections), and doesn't really solve the patient's problem. Guess who is likely to be paid more money under fee-for-service.

Outcomes and Alternatives

The system we need would be designed to produce favorable health outcomes efficiently. It would systematically gather data on treatments, resource use, and health outcomes (did the patient survive six months? did the treatment solve the problem? can the patient walk? work?). Clinical decisions would be based on analyses of such data. Dr. Paul Ellwood, a leading health-policy thinker, calls this "outcomes management."

The system we have knows little of outcomes data, virtually nothing of the relationship of resource use to outcomes. The scientific information base underlying much medical practice is small. For most medical treatments doctors simply cannot point to good relevant data linking outcomes, treatments, and resource use to support their choice of therapy in comparison with other reasonable but less costly alternatives.

Prevention and Follow-Up

The system we need would emphasize prevention, early diagnosis and treatment, and effective management of chronic conditions to prevent them from becoming serious acute problems. For instance, it would use computers to send reminders to parents of children scheduled for immunizations—and follow up until the children were immunized.

The system we have does poorly on prevention and primary care. Roughly 40% of children aged 1 to 4 lack basic immunizations for childhood infectious diseases. The US was down to 2,800 measles cases in 1985, but up to more than 18,000 by 1989. About 20% of white mothers and 40% of black mothers don't get prenatal care in the first trimester of pregnancy. But the US system is quite open to the financing of very costly high-tech care, such as neonatal intensive care for low-birthweight babies.

Total Quality Management

The system we need would practice "Total Quality Management/ Continuous Quality Improvement," the powerful management philosophy developed by W. Edwards Deming, Joseph Juran, and Philip Crosby that has led to the major gains in quality and productivity that we associate with world-class industrial competitors like Honda, Hewlett-Packard, and Xerox. The health services industry is virtually untouched by this movement. Only in the late 1980s did a few leading health-care organizations, such as the Harvard Community Health Plan and Intermountain Health Care, get seriously committed to continuous quality improvement. Health-care leaders such as Intermountain's Brent James and Harvard's Donald Berwick have made an impressive case that Continuous Quality Improvement could generate significant annual productivity improvements. *The system we have* violates modern concepts of quality management in many ways. It works on what Dr. Berwick calls "the bad apples theory." If a bad outcome happened, it must have been because some bad person messed up, and the system should find and penalize him. Not surprisingly, this attitude leads to coverups and evasion of accountability. *The system we have* doesn't embody proper statistical thinking. It looks at one case at a time to see what went wrong, rather than, say, 500 cases at a time to see what correlates with good outcomes. Physicians are socialized to have a self-image as autonomous actors whose correct decisions will save the patient. This works against the teamwork and process-mindedness, cutting across departments and professions, that is needed for Continuous Quality Improvement.

Selecting Doctors

The system we need would be based on organizations that carefully select doctors for quality and efficient practice patterns. Performance varies widely among physicians. Patients have a hard time assessing technical aspects of quality. That takes analysis of complex data from many patients. And most patients can't tell whether their doctor is up-to-date or not. They need systematic help.

The system we have has no effective mechanism to protect the population from poor or out-of-date doctors. Malpractice litigation doesn't separate the good from the bad. State regulators find they have to be able to prove unacceptable behavior in court to lift a medical license. The defendant doctors can tie them up in court for years, then move to another state.

Matching Doctors and Needs

The system we need would carefully match the numbers and types of doctors to the needs of the population served, with plenty of primary care physicians to assure patients convenient access to a doctor, and a number of specialists small enough to assure that each will have a full schedule seeing just the types of patients he or she was trained to see. This keeps the specialists proficient in their specialties and reduces their incentives to do unnecessary surgery.

The system we have has too many specialists and too few primary care doctors (general internists, family practitioners, pediatricians). The numbers and types of doctors turned out by residency programs are driven by the needs of government-subsidized training programs for cheap labor in the form of residents, and by student expectations of higher incomes and easier lifestyles in the specialties.

Economies of Scale

The system we need would concentrate complex procedures in high-volume regional centers to take advantage of economies of scale and experience. Research shows that, for complex operations like open-heart surgery, practice makes perfect: High volume is associated with low death rates and low costs.

The system we have proliferates facilities for heart surgery and other procedures—facilities that remain underutilized. In California, more than a third of the hospitals doing open-heart surgery have annual volumes below the 150 minimum needed for proficiency and patient safety. In Des Moines, Iowa, in 1987, one hospital did seven kidney transplants while another did ten. They should have been done at the University of Iowa Hospital, about 100 miles away, which handled 75 cases that year.

Making Technologies Prove Themselves

The system we need would put the burden of proof on expensive new technologies— and require their worth be proved before they are put in general use. It would conduct ongoing technology assessment and facilitate a rational response to the information produced.

In the system we have the courts, the media, and unrealistic patient expectations are forcing health insurers to pay for extremely costly technologies—such as autologous bone marrow transplants for AIDS —before they have been shown to be effective. Many very costly technologies are put into practice before they have been thoroughly evaluated.

Benefits Versus Costs

Finally, the system we need would encourage informed cost-conscious decision-making by doctors. They wouldn't do things having very high costs and very low marginal benefits. For example, Genentech has very successfully marketed TPA, a drug based on recombinant DNA technology, that dissolves blood clots diagnosed as causing heart attacks—for about $2,200 a treatment. Recent large-scale controlled trials show that intravenous streptokinaise is just as effective—at about $200 a treatment. Genentech's experts are debating the results. But TPA wouldn't sell much in a cost-conscious system.

Accountable Health Partnerships

How can Americans get from the system we have to the system we need? There isn't a simple single easy intervention that can get us there. We need a comprehensive strategy by *purchasers* that matches in sophistication the complexity of the *industry* we're trying to change.

Giving Power to Consumers

By combining individuals and employee groups into large purchasing cooperatives, managed competition creates a powerful, knowledgeable countervailing force on the demand side of the market. Health care has historically been characterized by strong providers and weak purchasers. Managed competition equalizes the relationship—indeed, the purchasing cooperatives will have an unprecedented capacity to restrain costs.

Paul Starr, *The American Prospect*, Winter 1993.

A group of health-policy analysts and industry leaders have been meeting annually at the home of Dr. Paul Ellwood in Jackson Hole, Wyoming, to discuss what such a comprehensive reform might look like. Here, in brief, are some of the main Jackson Hole Group proposals.

First, purchasers need to direct their purchasing to what Ellwood calls "Accountable Health Partnerships." These are defined as:

• Organizations that integrate the functions of care provision and insurance, so that providers share in the risks of the cost of care and are motivated to reduce cost.

• Organizations that are publicly accountable for quality and cost per capita using "generally accepted accounting principles" for outcome measurement and reporting (taking account of patient mix, for example).

• Organizations with greatly improved computerized clinical information systems that generate data relating outcomes to treatments and to resources used as a guide to improved medical practice.

• Organizations that can contract selectively with the numbers and types of doctors needed for the population served; that can select doctors and other providers; and that can contract at will (i.e., not renew contracts of poor performers without having to prove their deficiencies in court).

Standards Boards

American health care also needs a market-enhancing regulatory structure, comparable to what the Securities and Exchange Commission and the Financial Accounting Standards Board do for financial markets. Markets require information to function

175

effectively. The Jackson Hole Group proposes an "Outcomes Management Standards Board" to set data collection and reporting standards for Accountable Health Partnerships and to establish a national data system for patient outcomes and other quality measures.

Costly health technology decisions are now often being made irrationally by the courts and the media—who don't appear to understand why insurance companies should not be forced to pay for expensive therapies of unproven efficacy. Individual health plans and employers can't stand up to these pressures. They need help with such medical-lexicon decisions as: Under what conditions, if any, can patients benefit enough from liver transplants, autologous bone marrow transplants for metastasized breast cancer, and the like to justify the cost? These decisions must be made collectively by an informed authoritative process that can command respect and support. If the medical societies or insurance companies try to do it, they get sued for anti-trust violations.

The group proposes a "Health Standards Board" to assess medical technologies and medical practice effectiveness and advise on a list of "uniform effective health benefits" that would be covered by all tax-favored health insurance plans.

Next, consider that roughly half of American workers are employed in groups of 100 or less or are self-employed. These groups are far too small for the spreading of risk, for economies of scale in administrative costs, or for acquisition of the expertise needed to purchase health care effectively. Competition at the level of individual choice is blocked in small groups because such groups are not large enough to be able to offer competing health-care plans to employees. Employees in these groups need to be pooled into larger units. Richard Kronick, of the University of California, and I have proposed "Public Sponsors" and "Health Insurance Purchasing Corporations," collective purchasing agents for small employers and individuals.

Managed Competition

As it is, insurers often profit more from selecting good risks and segmenting markets than from joining with doctors to manage care efficiently, because the health-care market in general has not been structured appropriately. To correct this, I recommend to large employers and to Health Insurance Purchasing Corporations a strategy called "managed competition." Its purpose is to reward with more subscribers those health plans that provide high-quality care and effectively control cost, and to take the reward out of attempts to select risks and segment the market. The idea is to create a market driven by informed cost-conscious consumer choice.

176

Under this strategy, the large purchasers would:
- Qualify the competitors; preselect high-quality cost-effective comprehensive care organizations to participate.
- Run an annual open enrollment in which covered beneficiaries make choices and the health plans accept all comers.
- Structure prices to consumers so that consumers are fully price conscious in choice of plan; i.e., if Plan A costs $5 per month more than Plan B, those subscribers who choose Plan A pay $5 more.
- Contract for a standardized benefit package (list of covered services) to focus competition on total price and quality, not on whether Plan A offers birth-control pills while Plan B offers eyeglasses.
- Compensate the plans that enroll a disproportionate share of people with higher expected medical costs.

Market Forces

This all sounds pretty complicated. Why not just turn the whole US health-care system over to the government and let Washington run it? There are a lot of answers to that. I would be concerned by the possibility of a very large-scale replay of the Federal Savings and Loan and Federal Deposit Insurance Corporation fiascoes. Government can't pick good doctors or health-care organizations any more than it can pick good bankers. It can't create or order the system Americans need. I'd be concerned about the quality and economy of care produced by a government-run system.

But the answer I'd stress here is that we need to go from today's inefficient, wasteful system to a truly efficient one. And the only forces known to man that can transform inefficient industries into efficient ones are market forces. Government, especially the US government with all its checks and balances, just can't do that. What government might be able to do is help create a system of managed competition in which market forces take the health-care system from the one we have to the one we need.

177

"If what Americans want is more layers of bureaucracy micromanaging health care and generating red tape, managed competition is just what the doctor ordered."

Managed Competition Would Not Improve America's Health Care System

Judith Randal

Managed competition would be more expensive and would provide poorer health care than the current system or other alternatives, Judith Randal asserts in the following viewpoint. Randal maintains that allowing large health maintenance organizations (HMOs) to compete for patients will only increase the red tape that already burdens America's health care system. She concludes that the United States should adopt a system similar to systems used by many European countries, in which all citizens receive the same health care benefits and the government pays insurance companies to provide the care. Randal is a health and science writer who lives in Lovettsville, Virginia.

As you read, consider the following questions:

1. How might HMOs avoid covering chronically ill Americans under a system of managed competition, according to Randal?
2. Why does the author doubt that managed competition would save money?

From "Wrong Prescription: Why Managed Competition Is No Cure" by Judith Randal, *The Progressive*, May 1993. Reprinted by permission from *The Progressive*, 409 E. Main St., Madison, WI 53703.

A durable joke has it that the late Wilbur Cohen, an architect of Social Security and later Lyndon Johnson's Secretary of Health, Education, and Welfare, once asked God whether the United States would ever have national health insurance. "Only if I live long enough," God replied. If Congress does Bill Clinton's bidding by enacting the [president's] health-care reform plan, . . . the old joke will still be pertinent when the next election comes around. . . . It is no secret, however, that advocates of "managed competition" are calling the shots. . . .

The "managed" part of managed competition is shorthand for managed care. This means that patients would not select physicians for themselves, but would be enrolled in health-maintenance organizations (HMOs), and so would be locked in to the doctors who work for the HMOs and the hospitals and other facilities affiliated with them. (Preferred-provider organizations and independent-practice associations, while somewhat more flexible on this score, are variations on the same theme.)

The "competition" part of the formula means costs would presumably be kept down by having HMOs vie for customers. Large groups called health-insurance purchasing cooperatives would be set up to force HMOs to bid against each other on the basis of quality and price.

Logical as all this may appear on paper, the realities leave much to be desired.

Most of those who are now uninsured work for small businesses that insist they would go under—or at least resort to layoffs—if they had to provide the kind of health coverage paid for by big business. But big business, which is understandably indifferent to small-business concerns, generally favors managed competition. If times were good and the Federal treasury were flush enough to take much of the heat off small business (which is, after all, the nation's major source of new jobs), an accommodation could, perhaps, be reached. But under present circumstances, the best that can be expected from a managed-competition "solution" to the health-care crisis is an uneasy and temporary truce, with the needs of the public caught in the middle.

Poor Benefits

Under managed competition, consumers would have to pay more out of pocket for health-insurance premiums than most do now. And they would have to pay still more if they wanted fuller coverage than a mandatory basic-benefits package would provide—an option particularly important to parents of young children. Equally disquieting is that the benefits in the basic health-care package could well turn out to be stingier than those provided by many current policies.

There is still another possible bite on consumers: President

179

Clinton has talked of coupling "tax caps" to managed competition. This means that employers who agreed to a more generous—and hence more expensive—benefits package would not be able to deduct the entire cost as a business expense, as has always been permitted, but could only write off the cost equivalent of the basic package sold by the cheapest HMO in the area. And employees might be taxed for a portion of the heftier premiums as if they were a supplement to their wages, which would also be a first. Except for the self-employed, health-care premiums are now wholly tax-exempt.

What all this boils down to is that the lowest-cost HMOs, covering the fewest contingencies, would likely prevail. Managed competition would work well for the relative few with the means to buy top-dollar coverage, but it would weigh heavily on those who could afford it least—those with more than routine medical needs.

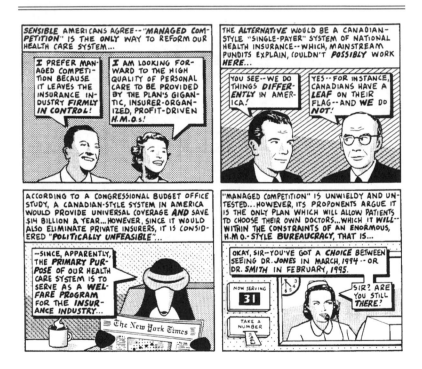

© 1993 Tom Tomorrow. Reprinted with permission.

The Clinton Administration is pledged to outlaw the now common denial of coverage on the basis of poor health or previous claims. The catch is that such a law is easily evaded. Insurers might refuse to contract with HMOs operating in zip codes where AIDS, tuberculosis, cancer, or other serious illnesses were prevalent. Or HMOs could keep the poor and disabled from their doors by setting up shop in places inaccessible by public transportation. Or HMOs might see to it that their physician turnover rates were high; the longer a physician practices in the same location, the more chronically ill patients he or she tends to accumulate.

Managed Competition Is Unlikely to Save Money

It isn't likely that managed competition can be counted on to save money. For one thing, at least two managed-care setups must be present in a community if there is to be competition, and each of them needs a potential market of roughly 250,000 people to achieve economies of scale. Only about half of all Americans, it turns out, live in places densely populated enough to support two or more such programs. What's more, insurers would constantly hustle to win and retain business, because employers would constantly be shopping for better deals, just as they do now. The sales staff, recruiters, advertising personnel, and clerical staff that such "marketing" entails contribute nothing to the provision of health care.

Moreover, large insurers could afford to spend more on marketing than smaller ones. The bigger the insurer, the greater the likelihood that consumer satisfaction would be a secondary concern.

And the physicians, nurses, and others whom insurers and HMOs hire to oversee—that is, second-guess—the decisions individual doctors make with individual patients—an essential feature of managed care—have to be paid, too. They tend to fuel hassles that generate paperwork and fray tempers all around, besides adding to the overhead cost.

Administrative costs already soak up about $225 billion a year—twenty-five cents of every dollar spent on health care in this country. Under managed competition, such costs would, at best, stay the same. More probably, they would increase.

Then there is the problem of co-payments and balance billing. The first is an additional charge many HMOs, preferred-provider organizations, and independent-practice associations impose on patients for actually rendering health-care services. Balance billing is the out-of-pocket expense faced by PPO, IPA, and some HMO patients if they seek care from physicians unaffiliated with their plans— the difference between the discount prices that these plans impose on their physicians and the higher fees independent doctors charge. Other HMO subscribers who obtain care from unaffiliated practitioners have to foot the entire bill themselves. Both mechanisms serve as escape hatches from cost constraints.

Far from being a new idea, managed competition is just another name for the prepaid health plans that were championed by the Nixon Administration in the 1970s, enabling it to fend off more comprehensive reform proposals then pending in Congress under Democratic sponsorship. What began as a trickle almost twenty years ago has since gained so much momentum that about 65 per cent of the insured population's care is already "managed" to at least some extent. Accordingly, the savings, if any, should be obvious by now.

Yet in the states where managed-care plans have the largest market share—Minnesota, Massachusetts, and California, for instance—health costs are no lower than in many other states and higher than in some. Prepaid-plan premiums in general have been rising just as fast as those for conventional "indemnity" policies that permit patients to see whatever physicians and go to whatever hospitals they choose without financial penalty. Small wonder, then, that even the Congressional Budget Office—usually one of President Clinton's favorite authorities—has its doubts as to whether managed competition would curb health-care expenditures by as much as its proponents claim.

A Faceless Health-Care System

Stripped to its essence, managed competition would complete the transformation of American medicine from one-on-one doctor-patient relationships to a medical system controlled by enormous, faceless corporate entities. It would establish a highly bureaucratic health-care system that would deprive patients of their ability to choose doctors and hospitals.

Advocates of managed competition would force most patients into huge HMOs run by insurance giants. Anyone who wants better care than the "minimum benefits package" would face steep financial penalties. Many who now have first-rate insurance plans would suddenly find themselves forced into cut-rate-type HMOs.

Nowhere in the world is there a working model of managed competition. It has never been tried. However, evidence suggests that strategy will not hold down costs. The past decade has seen enormous growth of HMOs and of managed care programs, at the same time that health costs have risen at record rates.

Business and Society Review, Winter 1992.

Theoretically, it is possible to restrain both health-insurance premiums and providers' charges for services by imposing a global health-care budget—a lid on total health-care spending.

But given not only the multiplicity of players, but also American medicine's unquenchable thirst for high technology, such a ceiling would be difficult to enforce.

The nation already has more mammography machines, open-heart surgery suites, magnetic-resonance imagers, and other big-ticket items than can be used efficiently, and they are often paid for by excessive charges and overuse. But if a facility lacks mega-gadgetry that its competitors have, it soon loses business. So it's a safe bet that despite the waste, high tech would continue to proliferate. In this sense, competition and managed care are conflicting goals.

In short, if what Americans want is more layers of bureaucracy micromanaging health care and generating red tape, managed competition is just what the doctor ordered. But if they want affordable insurance that leaves them free to choose their physicians and hospitals no matter where they live and where or whether they work, they need a system that empowers them rather than enriching the medical-industrial complex and health insurers (particularly those that own and operate networks of HMOs).

Problems with Canada's Plan

Canada's "single-payer" plan—so called because only one insurer, the government, pays the bills—has been highly touted as a desirable alternative to managed competition/managed care. In the context of the current debate, however, single-payer looks like a nonstarter, if only because it would put the health-insurance industry out of business—an unlikely eventuality, given that industry's powerful lobby. Besides, while the United States now spends more of its gross domestic product on health care than any other country, Canada ranks number two.

A better alternative—already tested in decades of real-life operation—is available, if only people searching for a solution to the nation's health-care crisis will stop ignoring its existence. One version or another of this "statutory" model is in place in Austria, Belgium, France, Germany, Japan, Switzerland, and the Netherlands.

In these systems, health insurance is under the social-security umbrella and is funded by payroll taxes or premiums that are set by law, as is a standard set of benefits that the entire population enjoys, regardless of age, health, income, and employment status. The money flows to private-sector health insurers or, as they are called in some countries, sickness funds. Individuals decide which of these nationwide plans they want to sign up with. When the insured or their dependents see a physician or go to a hospital, the bills are paid by that carrier. Choice of doctor and hospital is up to the patient.

The arrangement not only keeps commercial insurers in busi-

183

ness, but also has two other advantages. One is that it applies to everyone, so it eliminates the need for separate health-insurance programs for the elderly and the disabled (Medicare) and for the poor (Medicaid), both of which put their beneficiaries at a disadvantage because they pay doctors and hospitals less than do private insurers, and one of which (Medicaid) has a benefit package that varies from state to state.

Under a statutory model, it would not be necessary to resort to the kind of rationing scheme Oregon is adopting for Medicaid: denying some kinds of treatment to people now covered by the program to make it possible to include others who have no coverage at all. While European statutory insurance also has gaps in coverage, they do not apply only to the poor and those of modest means; in fact, they primarily affect the affluent, who can best afford to fill them on their own. In this country, it is the other way around, and would continue to be under managed competition.

What the Germans Do

The second major advantage of the statutory model is that it can be crafted to act as a brake on costs without the regulatory headaches that a global budget—a single, nationwide health kitty—would entail, even assuming that Congress would enact one and that it could be successfully imposed. William A. Glaser of the New School for Social Research has spent the better part of his career looking firsthand at how statutory insurance systems function in Europe and is among those who believe they can be made to do the job.

Germany's system, for example, limits periodic increases in premium costs for employers and workers to the annual rate of increase of the average wage. With that as leverage, Germany's 1,100-odd sickness funds join forces with labor unions, employer groups, and other interested parties to negotiate each year with hospitals and physicians' associations to keep their prices in line. In the five years from 1987 to 1992—a period when U.S. health-care expenditures soared upwards to the present 14 per cent of gross domestic product—health care's slice of the German GDP declined from 8.7 to 8.1 per cent.

Could the United States have such a system? Managed-competition proponents say no, insisting that the public wouldn't like it and the medical profession wouldn't put up with it. This country, they argue, is unique and therefore should have a system that is uniquely its own.

Perhaps. But if the Government decides that managed competition fills the bill, it will be less a system than an ideological fixation. Instead of curing what ails U.S. health care, it will leave it chronically ill.

"Universal health care is neither feasible nor plausible without health care rationing."

Rationing Health Care Is Effective and Necessary

Daniel Callahan

Daniel Callahan is director and cofounder of the Hastings Center in Briarcliff Manor, New York. The center is highly regarded for its research concerning biomedical ethics and health care issues. In the following viewpoint Callahan, a respected medical ethicist who has written numerous articles, explains his support for rationing health care—that is, limiting the type of medical procedures patients can receive. Currently, Americans are often able to choose expensive and sometimes unnecessary or futile medical treatments. This must end, Callahan states, for health care costs to decrease.

As you read, consider the following questions:

1. Why do other nations ration health care, according to Callahan?
2. What does Callahan think of Oregon's plan to ration health care? How is Oregon's plan different from other popular proposals to reform the health care system?
3. What questions must be addressed before adequate health care can be provided to all Americans, in the author's opinion?

From "Symbols, Rationality, and Justice: Rationing Health Care" by Daniel Callahan, *American Journal of Law and Medicine*, vol. 18, nos. 1 & 2, 1992. Reprinted with permission.

One of the most important domestic tasks before the United States is to put in place a just and universal health care plan. Most people seem to believe, however, that such a plan would obviate the need for rationing health care, indeed that it is an alternative to rationing. This [viewpoint] argues that universal health care is neither feasible nor plausible without health care rationing. This contention is based not on some theory of just health care but on the experience of other countries that have some form of universal health insurance already in place. Each provides a decent level of health care. None provide all the health care that people might want, nor necessarily provide it in the way in which they would most like to have it.

Why do these countries set such limits? Because early on they came to recognize what might be called the economic iron law of universal health care plans: to be affordable they must be limited. If you want universal coverage, then be prepared to ration. If you are not prepared to ration, abandon all hopes of an affordable plan of universal coverage. To these general propositions, good for all countries and times, must be added a specifically American point: if we ever hope to persuade American politicians to enact a plan of universal coverage, then we must show them in advance how such a plan will control costs and how it will have built into it the ingredients to keep it from breaking the bank. . . .

Oregon's Plan for Rationing

The Oregon initiative is of great national importance. Using a combination of technical and economic considerations, and tempering them with expressed public values, that state has set up a system of priorities. The Oregon legislators determined that it is better to provide health care coverage to everyone falling below the federal poverty line than to eliminate some people altogether in order to give virtually unlimited care to those who qualify. To make the new system possible, Oregon plans to limit services by means of its priority list. The plan will also mandate that small businesses provide health insurance or pay into a pool that would make that insurance available to all employed persons. The long-term goal is a system of universal health care in Oregon. [Oregon assigned a cost-effectiveness rating to 709 medical treatments, and plans to provide universal coverage for the top 587 of these. The list could be cut further. On March 19, 1993, Health and Human Services secretary Donna Shalala waived national Medicaid standards and approved the Oregon plan.]

As the Oregon planners recognized, any process of rationing health care will have to find a way to balance medical judgment, economic possibilities, and public values. Yet it took some years to gain that insight. When the Medicaid program was established by Congress in 1965 to provide health care for the poor, it specified that the indigent were to receive care that was "medically necessary." Congress did not, unfortunately (but perhaps deliberately) specify what that term meant or what means would be appropriate to make such a determination. It may have presumed that a purely medical standard of medical necessity could be determined.

Rationing Would Improve Access to Care

The present system of health care in the United States, with its explosive increases in costs and growing numbers of uninsured, is both unfair and financially unsupportable over the long run. As a result, policymakers will be looking increasingly at the option of rationing and the decisions it requires about the allocation of resources between low-technology primary care and high-technology specialty care. On balance, virtually all rationing schemes would make primary care more accessible than it is now.

Joshua M. Wiener and Raymond J. Hanley, *The Brookings Review*, Fall 1992.

If that is what Congress believed, it was wrong. As the intervening years have demonstrated well, it has turned out to be impossible to specify a purely scientific standard of medical "need," the basic concept that lies behind the idea of that which is "medically necessary." The problem is that "need" admits of no precise definition, ranging as it does over mental and physical needs, life-saving and life-enhancing needs. It is a notion, moreover, that is subject to different interpretations, open to the changed possibilities provided by technological developments, and subject to different valuative interpretations. Thus although "medically necessary" and meeting health care "needs" have about them the ring of objectivity, they turn out to be flexible and malleable concepts. They combine both a descriptive and a normative content. They are at once scientific and moral concepts. This was not so obvious in 1965.

How Much Care Is "Medically" Necessary?

As time has gone on, it has been possible to trace a steady enrichment of our understanding of the ingredients necessary to specify a decent minimum of adequate health care. Such care must include, in some plausible way, first, some reference to medical need; it must be rooted in commonly accepted notions of what people characteristically look for in health care. Yet, for all the above-mentioned reasons, it cannot use such a standard exclusively. Inevitably, many questions about the extent of those needs and the various evaluations required to deal with the borderline cases will arise. Second, therefore, a decent minimum of average health care must include judgments about the efficacy of available treatments to meet those needs; that is, what works and what does not work? A consideration of efficacy will, however, force a third set of considerations—that of the relative costs and benefits of different treatments. What will it cost to provide different benefits and is there a good return on the money spent?

Next a decision will have to be made. If not everything can be afforded, what treatments and benefits are relatively more or less important? At this point, it should be abundantly clear that this question and those that preceded it require a central political component to be properly answered. Because these questions address fact and value, and the weighing of costs and benefits, they transcend a technical level. The questions call for collective judgment, judgment of a kind that will combine both expert and lay opinion. Thus, the fourth consideration is that a political process will have to be devised.

Since the political process almost certainly will encounter resource limitations, a question will then be raised: what is relatively more or less important in the provision of health care? The setting of priorities, then, will be a fifth consideration. How might that best be done? The state of Oregon has devised one method to do this, and perhaps one could imagine others. Whatever other possible ways they might use to set priorities, however, other states would be wise in following the lead of Oregon in organizing community discussion of health care policy prior to the more formal political process of priority setting. Thus, the sixth consideration is the importance of giving the public not only a chance to express its opinions and preferences on priorities, but also a chance to become educated on the issues.

Rationing Will Completely Change the System

In a sharp attack on the Oregon approach to rationing and priority-setting, one of our most astute health care analysts, Lawrence D. Brown, wrote that "rationing has been elevated to the pantheon of fashionable solutions—competition, managed care, prudent purchasing, and more—that policymakers intermittently embrace as all-American answers to uncontrollable health care costs." He then goes on to say that

> [v]iewed in cross-national context, Oregon's contribution is mainly to show that, at least today in the United States, rationing is not a profound but a spurious issue. . . . The United States should worry less about rationing and more about constructing a rational policy framework whose watchwords are budgeting, planning, regulation, and negotiation. If the polity has declined to make those hard choices, rationing cannot

save it from itself. American policymakers have not earned the right to ration health care, and the very policies that would earn it would eliminate much of the need to exercise it.

Dr. Brown is wrong. First, rationing has not been proposed as one more solution to be put alongside competition or managed care, but as a strikingly different kind of proposal. The other approaches were all designed to control costs within the present system of health care, not to change the system altogether. For many, in fact, they were meant as ways of avoiding rationing, as rationing is a generically different kind of approach. Second, what Dr. Brown proposes is perfectly sensible, but it *also* is fashionable. For what has been more common of late than to call for "a rational policy framework," and the national health insurance that would embody it? It is the best solution, and even those of us who support rationing would prefer such a framework as our starting point in an ideal world. But Dr. Brown neglects to mention that there has been no national progress of any significance toward that goal. There has been neither the political will for such a framework nor, in the face of budget deficits, any serious, politically potent constituency for it.

Third, the real genius of the Oregon initiative is that it starts with a recognition of limits as the first step toward a comprehensive health care system. Its organizers say that in the present American political climate, the best way to get to Dr. Brown's goal of "budget, planning, and negotiation" is to concede at the very outset that rationing is necessary, and that the setting of priorities is the most sensible way of effecting it. It is striking that none of the major national universal health care plans that have been proposed make any serious provision for controlling their costs. The Oregon plan takes limitation as its *point of departure* and then works from there.

Oregon Is Making Progress

In effect, the Oregon plan stands Dr. Brown's approach on its head. Dr. Brown says that "American policymakers have not earned the right to ration health care, and the very policies that would earn it would eliminate much of the need to exercise it." The organizers of Oregon's plan, by contrast, say that only by a willingness to embrace rationing—the orderly, equitable allocation of scarce resources—can we make progress toward universal health care, not the other way around. They also say, moreover, that it is high time we stop talking about how a better, more rational system would obviate the need for rationing. No universal health care system could avoid some degree of rationing. In any case, we are still far from significant national reforms, and the need now is to find a good starting point. In the absence of the will, leadership and public support necessary for national health insurance, Oregon is actually taking some real steps in that direction. The other states and the federal government are just talking.

The animus against rationing in the United States, symbolically and literally, expresses in one sense some of our most admirable values. Those are our touching faith in the power of efficiency, our commitment to egalitarianism, and our reluctance officially to pick upon the poor to test our social schemes. Rationing is thought to offend all of those values and thus is rejected.

The Dream and the Reality

We deceive ourselves. Serious efficiency would require the equivalent of rationing, and that is why we have not achieved it. Our egalitarianism is more rhetorical than it is real. We tolerate a radically inegalitarian health care system as a day-to-day affair but then rail against anyone—in the name of perfection—who would accept some degree of inequality as the first step on the way to a genuinely fair system. Although we carry out social experiments with the poor all of the time, including the crazy mess that is our Medicaid system, we rail at efforts to bring some sensible priorities and planning into that system, as Oregon is trying to do.

The usual approach to American problems is to say that since we are such a powerful and rich nation, we can afford nothing less than the best: the most lavish health care system and, with reform, the fairest and most efficient as well. So we reject any notion of limits, boundaries or self-restrictions. We live with our dreams We should give them up and put realism and sobriety in their place. An acceptance of rationing would be a good place to begin. In fact, if we want national health insurance, it is likely to be the only feasible place to begin.

"Once you put a price tag on a person's life, inevitably it will be marked down."

Rationing Health Care Is Inhumane and Unethical

Nat Hentoff

Physicians have the duty to care for all patients who desire treatment, regardless of the seriousness of their illness, the expense of a procedure, or the chance of recovery, Nat Hentoff asserts in the following viewpoint. Rationing health care, he believes, would be inhumane and unethical, for it would prohibit physicians from treating patients who have little chance of recovery or who require expensive procedures. Hentoff maintains that because all lives are valuable, all Americans have the right to whatever health care they need and desire. Hentoff is a columnist for the *Washington Post* and the *Village Voice* newspapers, and a well-known commentator on social and political issues.

As you read, consider the following questions:

1. How will the poor be affected if health care is rationed, according to Hentoff?
2. Why does the author disagree with the argument that a patient's "quality of life" should be considered?
3. Why do some Americans support rationing health care, in Hentoff's opinion?

From "A Health Plan That Kills the Undeserving Poor" by Nat Hentoff, *The Village Voice*, September 22, 1992. Reprinted with the author's permission.

191

So have we decided that if a person has less than a 10 per cent chance of living for five years, that's it! The person's life is over?
—David Robison, an AIDS patient with less than a 10 per cent chance of living for more than five years—protesting Oregon's medical rationing plan that would remove him from the Medicaid rolls

[The Oregon rationing plan] *was an honorable choice, made with astonishing harmony by Republicans and Democrats.*
—Lead editorial, *The New York Times*, August 6, 1992

The Oregon plan rationed health care only for poor people enrolled in Medicaid. It appeared that poor women and children— those with the least political power—were required to bear the burden of controlling health costs.
—Robert Pear, *The New York Times*, August 5, 1992 . . .

Currently, a very popular approach among many doctors— and particularly among state officials with diminishing budgets—is to ration health care paid by Medicaid. A much admired pioneering model has been the Oregon plan. . . . Bill Clinton thinks the Oregon plan is just dandy. . . . Vice President Al Gore is opposed to the Oregon plan, and he correctly emphasizes that the continuing debate over this approach to rationing health benefits is "the single most important debate on the future of health care in the United States."

Excluding People from Care

Will government—federal, state, and local—be allowed to use a utilitarian measure—the greatest good for the greatest number—to decide who gets care and who doesn't? The Oregon plan lists 709 medical procedures and ranks them on the basis of their costs—and their benefits.

If a treatment is too costly in that it is not likely to sufficiently "improve" the patient's condition or is of insufficient value to society—then it will not be paid for. Of that list of 709 medical procedures in Oregon, everything below No. 587 would no longer be paid for.

In the years ahead, if the state budget gets leaner, the cutoff number for benefits will get lower. As of now, there would be no treatment, for example, for viral pneumonia, viral hepatitis, and chronic bronchitis.

Consider David Robison, quoted above. He has AIDS, and has developed cancer. According to the statistical averages, he has a more than 90 per cent chance of dying within the next five years. Robison would be on Line 688 of the Oregon plan.

Remember, we're dealing here with Medicaid, the combined federal-and-state financing for the poor. Oregon and its champions say that the plan brings 120,000 poor people—with no previous medical benefits—into Medicaid. What they don't say as loudly is that the state, to pay for these newcomers, is going to have to cut off other poor people who already received benefits before the lethal list of allowable medical conditions was promulgated. But if those already covered by Medicaid develop conditions below No. 587, they're out of luck and life. So are the newcomers.

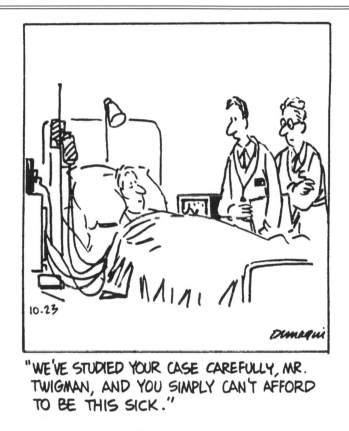

"WE'VE STUDIED YOUR CASE CAREFULLY, MR. TWIGMAN, AND YOU SIMPLY CAN'T AFFORD TO BE THIS SICK."

Reprinted with special permission of North America Syndicate.

Under this plan—predictably championed by President Bill Clinton—the poor are pitted against each other while the bureaucrats decide which of the poor shall survive. Another in the line of Jonathan Swift-like modest proposals to "take care" of the poor.

Said David Robison on the *MacNeil-Lehrer Newshour:* "I was raised to believe that if a person only has one day left to live, then that one day is very precious to that person and no other human being has a right to deny that person that one extra day of life."

Or, as Democratic congressman Henry Waxman of California, who is vehemently opposed to the Oregon plan, says: "Medical care should be based on the *individual*."

More in medical terms, William Schwartz, a professor of medicine at Tufts University, told *The New York Times:* "The expected value or payoff from any procedure depends on the particular characteristics and severity of an illness in a *particular patient.* Those variables are generally not reflected in Oregon's list of priorities."

David Robison's physician, David Regan, agrees with Schwartz—and goes further: "What if Robison has treatment, his disease put into remission, and a year from now a dramatic breakthrough occurs? . . . We can't turn our back on that group of patients. I think they have a right to try therapy before it's bureaucratically taken away from them.". . .

Determining Who Should Live or Die

The Oregon plan . . . is not only utilitarian. It was developed—as a supporter, Tim Ferguson, said in *The Wall Street Journal*—in a "communitarian" process.

In other words, if you lived in Oregon, a number of your fellow Oregonians, from various walks of life above poverty, would have helped determine whether you, if you were poor, deserved to be on Medicaid.

Commissions of the citizenry—business people, doctors, labor leaders—held 47 town meetings in the state to decide, in some instances, who would live and who would die under the plan. Then, believe it or not, there was a random telephone survey of 1000 Oregonians. They too became part of the business of deciding for other Oregonians whether their lives were worth saving with the taxpayers' money. . . .

"Quality of life," of course, is the terminating obbligato throughout the Oregon plan. If a treatment will make you normal again, then the society won't have to pay for repeated treatments, so you get Medicaid. But if your "quality" of life is such that you're not likely to be able to jump out of bed and jog along with Bill Clinton, well, damn it, you're going to keep on burdening the taxpayers. Off the list!

A quotation I've had nearby for a long time comes from an 18th century German doctor, Christopher Hufeland. A professor of medicine, he was a humanist and wrote on Goethe and Herder as well as on medical conditions. This is what he said, and it goes entirely counter to the Oregon rationing plan:

"If the physician presumes to take into consideration in his work whether a life has value or not, the consequences are boundless and the physician becomes the most dangerous man

194

in the state."

Some years ago, in Pennsylvania, a lively woman gave me what she said was an ancient folk saying:

"Once you put a price tag on a person's life, inevitably it will be marked down."

Not only marked down for a particular individual but also eventually for those throughout the society who have to depend on the state for health care. . . .

Supporters of the plan are essentially elitists. They themselves do not need Medicaid to get their health care. And so they are willing to let some of the poor be lopped off Medicaid to give room to others of the poor. If President Clinton allows this kind of plan to spread across the country, there will be no real national health insurance. It's easier to save money on the undeserving poor.

Periodical Bibliography

The following articles have been selected to supplement the diverse views presented in this chapter.

American Journal of Law & Medicine	Entire issue on "Implementing U.S. Health Care Reform," Vol. XIX, Nos. 1 & 2, 1993. Available from Membership Director, American Society of Law & Medicine, 765 Commonwealth Ave., Boston, MA 02215.
American Journal of Law & Medicine	Entire issue on "Rationing Health Care: Social, Political, and Legal Perspectives," Vol. XVIII, Nos. 1 & 2, 1992.
American Medical News	October 11, 1993. Special issue on health care reform. Available from 515 N. State St., Chicago, IL 60610.
Stuart M. Butler	"Have It Your Way: What the Heritage Foundation Health Plan Means for You," *Policy Review*, Fall 1993.
Philip Caper	"Managed Competition That Works," *Journal of the American Medical Association*, May 19, 1993. Available from Subscriber Services Center, American Medical Association, 515 N. State St., Chicago, IL 60610.
William A. Glaser	"The United States Needs a Health System Like Other Countries," *Journal of the American Medical Association*, August 25, 1993.
John Immerwahr et al.	"Whither Health Care Reform? A Roundtable," *Issues in Science and Technology*, Fall 1992.
Desmond Morton	"Health Insurance in Canada," *Dissent*, Spring 1993.
National Forum	Summer 1993. Entire issue on "Health Care Policy in America."
The New American	November 1, 1993. Entire issue on health care.
Steven G. Post	"Health Care Rationing?" *America*, December 5, 1992.
Reason	March 1992. Special issue on health care.
Tom Rother	"Rich, You Live; Poor, You Die," *New Unionist*, No. 193, August 1993.
Paul Starr	"Healthy Compromise," *The American Prospect*, Winter 1993.
Rachel Wildavsky	"Here's Health-Care Reform That Works," *Reader's Digest*, October 1993.

5 CHAPTER

Would Increased Regulation Improve the Health Care System?

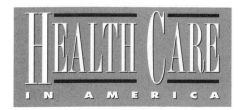

Chapter Preface

Federal, state, and local governments are key players in America's health care system. Medicare and Medicaid, health care plans for the elderly and the poor respectively, are just two of the numerous programs regulated by the U.S. federal government. State governments regulate the licensing of physicians and other health care professionals. Local governments often control funding to public hospitals, among other responsibilities. Such government regulation of health care divides Americans into two camps: those who believe government regulation protects consumers and those who believe it harms consumers by harming the economy.

Opponents of government regulation argue that the paperwork and bureaucracy that accompany government involvement prevent businesses from growing and contributing to the nation's prosperity. They also believe some requirements are unfair and counterproductive. For example, many object to President Bill Clinton's proposal that the government require businesses to provide health care benefits to their employees. Conservative writer William P. Hoar opposes such a move: "When government mandates additional job benefits (such as health coverage that many companies have simply not been able to afford), that increases the cost of labor and eats into profits. When workers become too expensive to keep on the payroll, employers lay off their employees or don't hire them in the first place." To Hoar, increased government regulation means decreased job opportunities and a depressed economy.

But Clinton and others disagree, arguing that by requiring businesses to provide health care benefits to employees, the government is protecting citizens, not harming them. "A lot of people agree with the concept of shared responsibility between employers and employees, and that the best thing to do is to ask every employer and every employee to share that," Clinton states. "The Chamber of Commerce has said that, and they're not in the business of hurting small business. . . . Every employer should provide coverage, just as three-quarters do now." Proponents believe that government regulation can protect citizens from unfair employers and from the threat of being uninsured.

The government can potentially regulate a broad range of health care services from vitamin manufacturers to insurance companies. The following chapter presents arguments supporting and opposing government regulation of the health care system.

"The health care crisis cannot be resolved without a radical change in the malpractice litigation system. "

Malpractice Awards Should Be Regulated

Jose Lozano

In the following viewpoint, Jose Lozano criticizes the malpractice litigation system in which physicians pay for malpractice insurance to cover possible lawsuits. Physicians are only human, the author states, and will make mistakes. It is unfair for patients to expect perfection from their physicians and unfair for courts to award huge amounts of money to those patients who do sue for malpractice. Besides, he notes, not every adverse outcome is the result of malpractice. The author concludes that the government must reform the malpractice system as part of its solution to the health care crisis. Lozano is an internist and nephrologist in private practice in Beaumont, Texas.

As you read, consider the following questions:

1. How does the author respond to the statement that "litigation is part of the American way of life"?
2. What are some of the consequences of the current malpractice system for physicians, according to Lozano?
3. How have advances in medical technology affected the way patients perceive medicine, in Lozano's opinion?

This country is facing a crisis in the delivery of health care services. . . . There is, however, significant disagreement on how to approach the search for the solution to this crisis.

The people in power do not always view the situation from the perspective of the millions of Americans without adequate health care access (30 million or more). The influential and powerful do not always start from the premise that health care is a basic human right, closely related to the preservation and protection of human dignity, and that adequate health care is not only the result of access to medical care, but also and very importantly, the product of other basic human rights, including employment, housing, education, food and clothing.

Until these philosophical concepts are adopted by this society, the United States will continue to provide the best available medical care in the world only for those who are able to pay, and the number of Americans without access to health care will continue to increase dramatically. More and more Americans will have to face the possibility of a major financial crisis as a result of illness.

The Threat of Lawsuits

Another important element of the health care crisis deserves further consideration. The health care crisis cannot be resolved without a radical change in the malpractice litigation system, which is having a profoundly negative effect on the delivery of health services. The practice of medicine, like other professions, is associated with a great deal of stress. In addition to dealing with pain, suffering and death on a daily basis, physicians face the threat of being sued for hundreds of thousands of dollars as a result of adverse medical outcomes. Although there are suits against other professionals, their total does not approach the aggregate of suits that have been filed against physicians.

Defensive medicine is a direct result of the malpractice system. It has been estimated that the cost of defensive medicine is approximately $20 billion per year.

Some argue that litigation is part of the American way of life, and that the malpractice system cannot be changed. However, the current system is having a tremendous impact on the life of physicians and on the quality of American health care. The public has been exposed to many anecdotal accounts of medical malpractice resulting from negligence. The public is unaware, however, that the litigation crisis is having a major effect on their medical care. The public has not been told that there are many situations in which doctors are the ones who suffer. Physicians may suffer major psychological trauma and financial stress as the result of the daily activities in the practice of medicine.

Sara Charles, MD, of the University of Illinois has extensively studied the impact of the malpractice system on physicians. She and others have identified a number of consequences, including: early retirement; changes in profession; changes in practice patterns, such as avoiding certain types of patients for fear of litigation; deterioration of the trusting relationship between patients and doctors; and a reduction in the joy of practice of medicine. The physician's mission is undermined by the idea that patients could potentially be a threat. It is difficult for a physician to understand that in today's society, litigation or potential litigation is a part of the daily practice of medicine and not a judgment of competence.

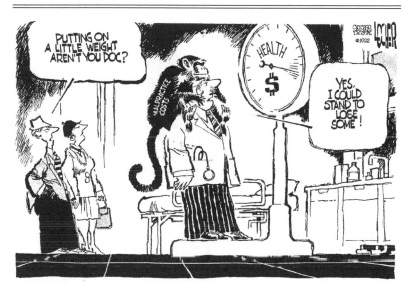

By permission: Tribune Media Services.

The final result is a decrease in the availability of and access to medical care for all members of the society. As indicated by Eugene Kennedy, co-author with Dr. Charles of the book *Defendant*, "This experience is draining the vitality of American doctors and . . . affecting everybody's health care."

Excessively High Expectations

In order to understand the complexity of the malpractice problem, certain psychological realities must be considered. Most people expect, on a deep unconscious level, that their physician will be perfect. Furthermore, in this highly technological society, there is a perception that everything can be fixed by an expert. The truth remains, however, that not every medical treatment or surgical operation can or will be successful. Both patients and physicians, like other human beings, are imperfect. L.M. Davey, MD, professor of neurosurgery at Yale University, maintains that "until society, which includes the courts, looks objectively at expectations in the field of health, the American civil justice system will remain as some have described—neither civil or just."

Many medications and procedures have unpleasant or undesirable side effects. Adverse outcomes are not always indicative of medical negligence. Physicians may arrive at the proper diagnosis and provide excellent medical care, and still obtain results that are less than perfect. Any bad medical outcome, including death, is not equal to negligence. Death, although undesirable, is unavoidable; without exception, it is the final act of human life.

Until true reform is undertaken, to be able to function effectively as a physician, it is helpful to keep in mind the observation of an independent insurance consultant from Houston, who wrote in the December 1990 issue of *Texas Medicine:* "I learned early that when the physician is sued with a malpractice, it signifies the death of the physician's naive belief that because he practices good medicine he is immune to this type of legal redress, it signifies the death of the illusion because he is a doctor . . . that patients all love him and would not dare sue him. . . . Welcome to the real world, Doctor!"

2 VIEWPOINT

"Malpractice reform would not result in significant savings in health-care costs. "

Malpractice Awards Should Not Be Regulated

Philip H. Corboy

Philip H. Corboy, a partner in the law firm of Corboy & Demetrio, represents plaintiffs in personal injury and wrongful death lawsuits. He is a former president of the Chicago Bar Association, former chairman of the Section of Litigation of the American Bar Association, and former president of the Illinois Trial Lawyers Association. In the following viewpoint, Corboy opposes increased government regulation of the malpractice system. Malpractice awards are not to blame for rising health care costs, he states, despite what many physicians argue. Corboy believes that the malpractice system is necessary and effective in punishing incompetent physicians and compensating injured patients.

As you read, consider the following questions:

1. Why does the author believe that caps on malpractice awards will not reduce physicians' malpractice premiums?
2. How is defensive medicine itself a form of malpractice, in Corboy's opinion?
3. Why is malpractice liability necessary, according to the author?

From "Medical Malpractice Insurance and Defensive Medicine" by Philip H. Corboy. Reprinted from *National Forum: The Phi Kappa Phi Journal*, vol. 73, no. 3, Summer 1993, © 1993 by Philip H. Corboy, by permission of the publishers.

From one vantage point, reforming health-care policy is no different from baking bread or building a house: what to leave out is as important as what to put in. In 1993 the American Medical Association (AMA) and the health-care industry embarked on a very public campaign to add tort "reform" to the Clinton administration's proposed health-care package. They propose saving Americans billions of dollars in health-care costs by reducing malpractice awards and eliminating "defensive medicine." Setting policy in this area is difficult because there is much that we do not know about how the legal system, insurance industry, and medical professions interact. However, we do know more today than we did during previous campaigns to "reform" the civil justice system. What we have learned indicates that limiting the rights of victims of malpractice will not cut costs. In fact, such an occurrence is likely to increase the national health-care bill while lowering the quality of our medical care.

Limiting Damage Awards

Tort "reform" encompasses a variety of legal changes designed to make it more difficult for injured victims to sue those responsible. These include shorter statutes of limitations, mandatory review of claims by other doctors or panels, a credit to a defendant doctor for money the plaintiff received from collateral sources, including health insurance, installment payments of awards, and various additional procedural devices. But the reform the medical-care industry wants most, by far, is a limit on the amount of money juries can award injured plaintiffs or the surviving spouses of deceased victims of malpractice. "Most doctors and hospitals say they prefer an outright cap on damage awards," reported the *Wall Street Journal* on 28 April 1993. The AMA's general counsel, Kirk Johnson, declared that a system that did not include damage caps "is not going to restrain costs."

There is a superficial appeal to this notion in political terms. What better way to win the support of the two most powerful special-interest groups in the field—doctors and insurance companies—than to offer a legal benefit they have sought for decades? Proponents are careful to portray damage limits not as a loss of the legal protections currently enjoyed by all Americans, but as a hit against trial lawyers. Actually, a certain amount of skepticism based on the financial interests of both the legal and the medical professions is healthy. But drastic changes affecting two areas of fundamental concern to Americans, their justice system and their health-care system, must not be imposed on the basis of rhetoric or interest-group politics. This is one decision that ought to be made on the facts. Can those who want malpractice reform added to the health-care package demonstrate that it will reduce the cost of health care for Americans while maintaining its quality? . . .

Before we embark upon major surgery on both our legal and health-care systems, we ought to look at the facts.

The fundamental message announced by [many] researchers is that the picture of our system of civil justice as "broken" or "out of control" is just not true. No one enjoys being sued, and there may be occasional cases—invariably spotlighted and distorted by the media—of the type President George Bush called "those crazy lawsuits." Overall, however, the system does what it was designed to do, imposes liability on negligent health-care providers for the damage they cause in a stable and predictable fashion. The Harvard Medical Practice Study of hospital medical records in allegedly litigious New York reveals that only one out of eight patients who was injured by negligence ever filed a claim. Juries find in favor of plaintiffs in only about one-third of cases, a far lower rate than in most other types of tort actions. Jury studies also indicate that the amount of damages awarded tends to reflect closely the victim's medical expenses. Moreover, appellate courts freely reduce or reverse awards that are not supported by the evidence.

HAGAR THE HORRIBLE by DIK BROWNE

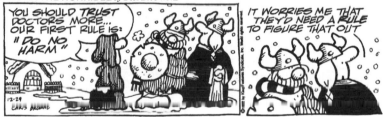

Reprinted by special permission of King Features Syndicate.

Perhaps the greatest significance of this empirical research lies in exposing the myth of the "lucky lotto plaintiff." The rationale for imposing a ceiling on damage awards is based entirely upon this myth. Proponents of reform are fond of portraying the tort system as a lottery in which a few lucky plaintiffs "strike it rich" by playing upon the sympathy of jurors. Capping damages, they assert, merely reduces the undeserved "profit" that some plaintiffs (and their lawyers) make from the system.

Researchers have not located the lucky plaintiff. Virtually every study of jury decision making demonstrates that jurors make their findings on the basis of the evidence in the case. Neither emotion nor sympathy interferes with their responsibility. Indeed, in finding liability and assessing damages, jurors tend to be at least as skeptical and conservative as judges or evaluators of professional claims looking at the same factual situation. If anything, victims with serious injuries tend to be the most unlucky category of plaintiffs. Large verdicts tend to involve brain damage or some other severely disabling injury that will require extensive medical care for many years, in addition to loss of income. Researchers for the Rand Corporation found that awards above $250,000, including amounts granted for pain and suffering, tend to be insufficient to cover actual economic loss. It seems that the higher the award, the greater the undercompensation. So many studies have confirmed this fact that Yale law professor Michael Saks concluded that "overcompensation at the lower end of the range and undercompensation at the higher end is so well replicated that it qualifies as one of the major empirical phenomena of tort litigation." Even if damage caps could result in lower health-care costs, it should be troubling that the entire burden is placed on those who are not only the more seriously injured victims but are also undercompensated under present tort law.

Faulty Assumptions

The assertion that limiting malpractice awards will reduce health-care costs contains three important assumptions. The first is that caps on awards for damages will save liability insurers a significant amount in lower claims payments. The second assumption is that the insurance companies will pass along these savings to doctors and hospitals in the form of lower premiums. Third, it is assumed that doctors will pass along lower malpractice premiums to their patients in the form of lower fees. In addition, proponents assume that tort reform will not actually add to the cost of health care in certain other ways. Specifically, there is no attention paid to terribly injured people who may now recover significant damages but who would be limited if caps were invoked. All of the assumptions must be true if Americans are to realize any savings. The fact is that each of these assumptions is unwarranted.

Capping Malpractice Awards Will Not Significantly Reduce Claims Payments. Americans spent more than $838 billion on health care in 1992. According to the AMA's own figures, premiums for medical malpractice insurance for hospitals and doctors totaled less than 1 percent of that figure. In other words, if insured malpractice suits were abolished entirely, the savings would represent less than 1 percent of America's health-care bill. For this reason, the Congressional Budget Office concluded that malpractice reform would not result in significant savings in health-care costs.

Limiting damages, of course, would affect only a small fraction of that 1 percent. A U.S. General Accounting Office survey of all medical malpractice claims conducted in 1984 revealed that less than 10 percent of payments exceeded $250,000. Less than 1 percent exceeded one million dollars. Only 5 percent of paid claims included noneconomic damages above $100,000. Studies in individual states confirm that large verdicts represent a very small fraction of the total number of malpractice suits.

Although a limit on damages has a devastating impact on severely injured individuals, the effect on total liability payments is minuscule. For this reason, both the Insurance Services Office, which advises the industry with respect to rates, and St. Paul Fire and Marine, the nation's largest medical-malpractice insurer, have publicly announced that caps on noneconomic damages would not lead to reduced insurance premiums. Indeed, in a number of states, including Indiana and California, enactment of a cap on damages was followed by sizable increases in rates.

Reduced Payments to Victims Will Not Result in Lower Malpractice Premiums. Even if tort changes significantly lowered the amounts that insurers paid to negligently injured plaintiffs, there is no reason to expect the carriers to pass along the savings to doctors. In most states, the malpractice-insurance market is dominated by a few carriers who are exempt from federal antitrust laws. Their customers have substantial incomes and need their product. . . .

Lower Malpractice Premiums Will Not Result in Lower Medical Costs. Although insurance premiums are a significant expense, they still represent only about 5 percent of the average gross income of doctors, approximately the same proportion that doctors paid in 1976. Any reduction in premiums, therefore, would not represent a significant reduction in expenses. . . .

Defensive Medicine

Some proponents claim that tort reform will also reduce health-care costs by eliminating "defensive medicine." This label has become a buzzword virtually devoid of meaning. The AMA asserts that a large percentage of physicians engage in practices that are motivated solely to avoid malpractice suits, rather than the medical needs of their patients. This is in itself malpractice! That any physician would admit to what amounts to unethical practice is astonishing. More revealing, however, are the practices these doctors consider defensive medicine: spending more time with patients, more thorough explanations of risks, more frequent consultations with other doctors, more follow-up visits, and additional testing. A great deal of defensive medicine strongly resembles good medicine.

The reformers focus on the use of unnecessary tests. A study released by the National Medical Liability Reform Coalition (NMLRC), which is lobbying for tort reform, estimates that adoption of a long list of reforms would eliminate $4.9 billion in defensive medicine during the first year. This number was based on a previous AMA estimate of the cost of defensive medicine that the NMLRC study admitted was "suspect" and possibly "overstated." Even if accurate, however, the saving would still be far less than 1 percent of total health costs.

The primary examples of defensive medicine cited in the study were electronic fetal monitoring and routine x-rays following minor head trauma, both of which were characterized as unnecessary in most instances. It is worth considering the relatively modest cost of these procedures compared with the risk of serious brain damage due to undetected fetal distress or intracranial injury. Apart from the human tragedy, the medical expense of caring for the victims of such often runs several hundred thousand dollars a year for life. Even if 99 percent of these procedures are unnecessary, avoiding even a small number of catastrophic injuries more than offsets their cost. . . .

Without Malpractice There Is No Malpractice Liability

Finally, there is the plain truth that the real cause of liability for medical malpractice is medical malpractice. Imposing liability for harm resulting from negligence is a powerful deterrent to negligence. Implicit in the argument concerning defensive medicine is the acknowledgment that the fear of malpractice suits makes doctors and hospitals careful. . . .

Behind the statistics are the faces of real people severely harmed by the negligence of those to whom they looked for health care. Those affected by caps have proved liability and damages in court. Often they are children suffering physical and mental deficits whose families face the prospect of a lifetime of medical expense simply to keep their children alive. What sort of justice is it to award such a family an amount that will run out after a few short years? One Kansas judge, striking down that state's damage cap as unconstitutional, condemned it as "economic euthanasia." A health-care policy that imposed such a heavy burden on a few unfortunate victims merely to provide a potential saving in health-care costs for society as a whole should present disturbing questions of conscience.

The facts, however, show that there would be no savings for Americans. If anything, the national medical-care expenditures are likely to increase while the quality of care declines. Most of the states have rejected damage caps, even in the face of alleged "crises." What we have learned demonstrates that there is no place for tort reform in a national health-care policy.

3 VIEWPOINT

"For the Mercks, Upjohns and Eli Lillys now to lean on their R&D as an excuse for price-gouging sends ample warning of what lies ahead."

The Price of Pharmaceutical Drugs Should Be Regulated

Lionel Van Deerlin

Pharmaceutical companies reap vast profits by overpricing drugs, Lionel Van Deerlin argues in the following viewpoint. He states that only by reining in this corporate greed can America reduce its health care costs. Van Deerlin advocates government regulation of the cost of pharmaceutical drugs. Van Deerlin, a former California congressman, is a columnist for the *San Diego Union-Tribune* newspaper.

As you read, consider the following questions:

1. How does the author respond to the drug companies' contention that high-priced drugs pay for research and development?
2. What did the late senator Estes Kefauver do to help cut the cost of pharmaceuticals, according to Van Deerlin?
3. How is the pharmaceutical industry fighting government regulation, according to the author?

"Adverse Side Effects" by Lionel Van Deerlin, *The San Diego Union-Tribune*, February 16, 1993. Reprinted with the author's permission.

Sometimes a complicated subject turns out to be simpler than anyone thought—if reduced to a few telling points we can all understand.

In opening his campaign for health care reform, President Clinton drew a bead on the drug industry. He noted that a polio vaccination priced at $1.80 in England costs nearly $10 in this country.

Response from the pharmaceutical lobby was immediate, its tone predictable. The following is from one news report:

"Drugmakers defended their prices as the product of research, development and legal protection costs. In 1990, the average R&D [research and development] cost for each new drug topped $250 million."

Oh? But wait a minute. The great Jonas Salk, whose historic polio vaccine scored the breakthrough against once dreaded infantile paralysis, carried out his research entirely on *public* funds at the University of Pittsburgh. This most celebrated drug research success of the 20th century bore no commercial logo.

For the Mercks, Upjohns and Eli Lillys now to lean on their R&D as an excuse for price-gouging sends ample warning of what lies ahead. Layer upon layer of huge private enterprises have formed a cocoon around U.S. health care—and they'll field a small army of lawyer-lobbyists bent on defeating any reform.

The cost of medical services has risen at a pace which is three times the cost of living generally. And elderly Americans, who need prescription drugs more often than any other segment of society, know the worst runaway has been at the pharmacy counter.

Moreover, regular Medicare covers no prescription drugs, and most supplemental insurance plans repay only a portion of these expenses.

Profit First, People Last

Now Clinton undertakes to show that the very youngest among us, as well as the oldest, are being shorted by a system that never has seemed to "put people first."

His is not the first effort to break the stranglehold. The late Sen. Estes Kefauver of Tennessee conducted a series of hearings which laid bare some surprising truths more than 30 years ago. It was revealed that countless patients, some at the edge of poverty, were paying many times what they should have done for certain drugs. This happened because doctors who might have ordered remedies by their "generic" name (denoting chemical content) instead prescribed by the fancy names given these same drugs under a commercial trademark.

Among the more egregious examples: Carter Wallace's Miltown was priced at $61.20 for 1,000 tablets, but under its generic name, meprobamate, the prescription cost only $4.95. Ciba's Serpasil carried a price tag of $49.50 per 1,000, though a matching supply of its generic equivalent, reserpine, could be obtained for $1.35.

Kefauver found that even government hospitals were being fooled—indeed, were wasting $750 million a year in public funds ordering drugs by trade name rather than generic designation.

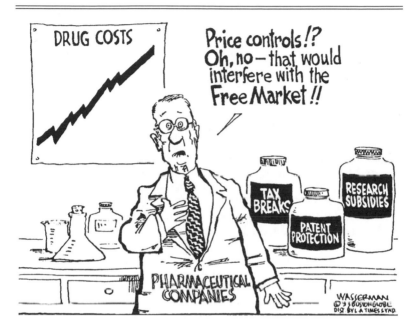

© 1993 Boston Globe. Distributed by Los Angeles Times Syndicate. Reprinted with permission.

Also targeted in Kefauver's legislative reform effort was the industry's failure to list on its labels the possibly undesirable side effects of certain drugs. The pharmaceutical lobby was well on its way to killing this provision until late 1962, when a succession of women who had used the drug thalidomide to ease child-bearing suddenly began delivering babies who were missing parts of arms or legs. Congress hastily enacted Kefauver's labeling requirements in even tougher form than the Tennessean had offered them.

The discrepancy between prices charged in the United States and other countries, for identical drug products, was brought to light by Wisconsin Sen. Gaylord Nelson. He heard from a resident of Sault St. Marie, Mich., who was paying $82.68 for 1,000 capsules of Upjohn's anti-diabetic Orinase. The man had then found the same product available in Sault St. Marie, Canada—just across the border—for $6.63.

Regulating Drug Prices

Like many nations, Sen. Nelson learned, Canada has a compulsory licensing system on drugs to protect its people against price gouging.

That revelation came more than 20 years ago. But as Bill Clinton now finds, nothing has changed.

The pharmaceutical lobby, operating out of two old-line Washington law firms (Covington & Burling, and Wilmer, Cutler & Pickering) remains at the battlements, ever ready to slow down regulatory orders and to discourage Congress in its oversight role.

Or, where these tactics fail, to take regulators to court.

In September 1968, a panel of the National Academy of Sciences reported some alarming findings about the drug Panalba, marketed by Upjohn. The scientists faulted this product in 110 documented cases of adverse results, including 12 deaths. The Food & Drug Administration moved to recall current stocks and bar further sales.

Stonewalling lawyers met rejection at every judicial level, including the Supreme Court. But their flood of litigation achieved what they really were after—delay. Panalba was not taken off the shelves until late March 1970, fully 1½ years after the scientific case against it had prompted the FDA's original order. No one can say how many additional victims this drug claimed while the legal arguments, and Upjohn's sales, went merrily on.

Bring medical costs down? Clinton has started out tough, but he'll have to keep the pressure on. Some equally tough and well-financed guys in pinstriped suits will be out to get him at every turn.

"A majority [of new drugs] did not even cover the companies' investment in research and development."

The Price of Pharmaceutical Drugs Should Not Be Regulated

Murray Weidenbaum

Murray Weidenbaum, a former advisor to the Reagan administration, is director of the Center for the Study of American Business (CSAB) at Washington University in St. Louis, Missouri. In the following viewpoint, Weidenbaum defends the prices pharmaceutical companies charge for their drugs. Drugs are expensive to discover, develop, and produce, he states. Regulating the price of drugs would not reduce health care costs and would only hurt Americans in the long run. Weidenbaum advocates increasing competition in the pharmaceutical industry to reduce the cost of drugs.

As you read, consider the following questions:

1. Why is developing a new drug such a lengthy and expensive process, according to Weidenbaum?
2. What statistics does the author cite to show that drugs are not overpriced?
3. How would consumers suffer from price controls, in the author's opinion?

From "Are Drug Prices Too High" by Murray Weidenbaum. Reprinted, with permission, from: *The Public Interest*, No. 108 (Summer 1993), pp. 84-89, © 1993 by National Affairs, Inc.

The American pharmaceutical industry is under assault. Patients are upset about the high prices of medicines. Congressional committees and consumer groups are aroused by reports of high profits. And the president of the United States has repeatedly promised to "crack down" on pharmaceutical companies, presumably through some form of price control.

Pharmaceutical companies have responded that drug costs make up only a small share of health-care costs, and that drug prices have risen no faster than other health-care prices. The companies also argue that the public's concern arises largely from the way health-care costs are financed: Many insurance and benefit programs, notably Medicare, do not cover prescriptions. As a result, prescriptions are paid largely out of pocket, and so come in for a disproportionate share of criticism.

These arguments, however valid, have failed to satisfy the public or its representatives. In the memorable words of Sen. Howard Metzenbaum (D-OH), "It is hard to believe that a company could charge so much for such a tiny pill." Such sentiments, when taken with the congressional tendency to legislate first and investigate later, make a closer look at medicine prices imperative.

Why It Takes So Long

It should be acknowledged at the outset that new drugs are sometimes very profitable. The U.S. Food and Drug Administration (FDA) does grant manufacturers patent protection (albeit for a limited time). But the other side of the coin is that the odds of coming up with a financial blockbuster are extremely low. A Duke University study of one hundred new drugs, for example, revealed that a majority did not even cover the companies' investment in research and development.

Why is profitability so elusive? The answer lies in the extended process of drug development and approval. On average, 5,000 different compounds must be tested for each drug ultimately approved by the FDA. Drugs must be tested in the laboratory, on animals, and on humans. A study at Tufts University reports that it takes an average of twelve years to get from initial research through FDA approval. . . .

Development Costs

Drug development is not only very time-consuming; it is also very costly. Studies at the University of Rochester, Texas A&M, and Tufts University show that the average cost of developing a new drug rose from $54 million in the 1970s to $125 million in the 1980s, and to $231 million in 1990.

A 1993 study by the congressional Office of Technology Assessment (OTA) reports that "a reasonable upper bound" on the full cost of R&D for a successful drug is $359 million (no "lower bound" was reported).

The basic incentive to make such investments is the possibility of high profits. As University of Chicago economist Sam Peltzman has pointed out: "Drug companies undertake these massive searches knowing there will be a big pay-off if they hit a winner. We can have lower drug prices if we accept less of that searching [for new chemical compounds]. That's the choice we face."

Rewards Are Necessary

The costs and risks of developing pharmaceuticals are so high that substantial rewards for success are necessary to motivate investment. These risks are not eliminated just because they are borne by large corporations that have survived precisely by being good at what they do. Destruction of those rewards will lead to erosion of the pharmaceutical industry's international competitiveness, a slowdown in new drug development, the perpetuation of less-effective and more-expensive treatments, and, ultimately, an intensification of the health care crisis.

The focus of the current debate on drug prices misses the point. This country has seen too many serious problems made worse by "quick fixes." The real question is how to ensure that pharmaceuticals continue to play a key role in improving the quality and cost-effectiveness of health care.

The Boston Consulting Group, Inc., *The Contribution of Pharmaceutical Companies: What's at Stake for America, September 1993.*

The consequences of that choice are on vivid display in Canada, where stringent price controls were imposed in 1969. In the two-and-a-half decades since, Canadian pharmaceutical companies have developed virtually no innovative medicines.

Similarly, Lacy Glenn Thomas of Emory University has found that countries like France and Austria, which have the toughest price restrictions on pharmaceuticals, also do the least research.

Not So Expensive

Critics of the pharmaceutical industry invariably ignore such points, and instead focus on the fact that prices have risen. Between 1985 and 1990, they point out, spending on pharmaceuticals rose from $20 billion to $32 billion. Yet what's not mentioned is that during this same period (and on through 1992), the cost of outpatient medicines held steady at 4.8 percent of total medical expenditures. In other words, the cost of drugs has risen at about the same rate as other health-care costs.

The price record prior to 1985 is also revealing. From 1966 to 1982, outpatient drugs were a steadily declining share of U.S. health-care expenditures—from a high point of 8.8 percent in 1966 to a low of 4.7 percent in 1982. We can only speculate as to why the improvement in the relative cost of drugs halted in the early 1980s. Perhaps the rapid rise in the cost of developing new drugs has played a part. We would expect that scientists would first discover and companies first market the medicines that are easiest to develop. Over time, the more difficult and expensive medicines would be brought to market.

Researchers have also pointed to some other reasons for price increases: the use of more patients in clinical trials, increasingly complex testing, and the growing interest in developing treatments for chronic and degenerative diseases like cancer and Alzheimer's.

Drug prices must also be seen in perspective. While many new drugs are expensive, they often enable patients to avoid painful and even more costly surgery. The cost of treating ulcers with H-2 antagonist drug therapy runs about $900 a year. The cost of ulcer surgery, by contrast, averages $28,900. . . .

Price Controls

Despite these facts, many people continue to believe that drug prices are far too high. The obvious way to lower them, it seems, is with price controls. Of course, the U.S. has had a great deal of experience with controls. There were general price controls during World War II, the Korean War, and the 1971 to 1973 period. Many municipalities continue controlling rents to this day.

The experience has been uniformly adverse. When faced with price controls, investors shift their funds to sectors of the economy without controls (as New York City's deteriorating housing stock reminds us). Consumers also suffer, because price controls create shortages. These shortages may be quantitative, as occurred in many markets from 1971 to 1973, or qualitative, as the Canadian drug market is suffering now. (In Canada, the availability of drugs developed in the U.S. has helped alleviate the problem. But American consumers would not have such a ready alternative.) . . .

More Competition

Fortunately, there is an alternative to price controls. That alternative is more competition. Of course, some careful consideration is necessary. Simply eliminating the patent protection enjoyed by developers of new drugs would not work.

What's needed instead is broader price competition. It could be encouraged in a number of ways. Many states, for example, now prohibit the advertising of prescription drug prices. These prohibitions make it difficult for consumers to shop for the best price. Such restrictions should be repealed. Even Sen. David Pryor (D-AR), a pharmaceutical industry critic, has urged that "any reform effort should make sure that both doctors and patients are more aware of prices."

At the federal level, the FDA should lower its advertising barriers. There need be little concern about deceptive advertising. Because consumers must first obtain prescriptions from physicians, there is less reason to fear deception in this market than in any other. The evidence, moreover, clearly shows that advertising can lower prices. Such evidence was cited by the Supreme Court in its decision overturning state bans on the advertising of eyeglasses.

The FDA's rules governing advertising are also needlessly bureaucratic. The agency should reconsider its requirement that a "brief summary" accompany any ad mentioning both a health condition and a drug treatment. The notorious "brief summary" is actually a lengthy statement listing side-effects and contraindications. Such information is essential for physicians, but incomprehensible to the average patient. More importantly, the "brief summary" requirement works to discourage advertising by making it needlessly cumbersome and expensive.

In Sum

There are several lessons here. The first is that while some drugs are very profitable, many more are not. The second is that price controls would be a mistake. The third is that what's needed is more competition. Warts and all, the competitive marketplace is the best protector of consumers.

"Employment-based health insurance . . . offers to policymakers a ready-made structure for achieving their objectives of universality and cost constraint."

Employers Should Be Required to Provide Health Insurance

David A. Rochefort

David A. Rochefort is an associate professor of political science and public administration at Northeastern University in Boston, where he was project administrator and coauthor of the report *Insuring American Health for the Year 2000*. He admits that employment-based health benefit programs have had flaws in the past, but he maintains in the following viewpoint that these flaws can be overcome. Examining and refuting many of the charges that have been brought against the concept of employer mandate insurance plans, Rochefort concludes that this would be the best model for health care reform.

As you read, consider the following questions:

1. What concerns about the economic impact of employer mandates does Rochefort address? How does he refute the arguments against mandates?
2. How does the author rebut complaints that employer-mandated insurance would be unfair to some workers and businesses?

From "The Pragmatic Appeal of Employment-Based Health Care Reform" by David A. Rochefort, *Journal of Health Politics, Policy, and Law*, Fall 1993. Copyright Duke University Press, 1993. Reprinted with permission of the publisher.

That employment-related health benefits have unjustly omitted many Americans from insurance coverage is easy to see. And current state-level public health insurance programs serving welfare recipients and the poor generally do not compare favorably with private insurance plans (except in the area of long-term care). But these points constitute more an indictment of *past* practices than a criticism of possible reforms. In fact, it is entirely feasible to design an employment-based health insurance program that would address such concerns, effectively marrying social justice with political pragmatism. To appreciate that such a program could be devised, however, it is necessary to set aside some major misconceptions about employer mandates that have entered into the national health policy debate.

A Crossfire of Criticism

Under a national employer mandate, the primary method for extending health insurance coverage would be to require all businesses to provide employees and their dependents with a standard basic package of benefits. Depending on the nature of this requirement, companies could do this directly or by paying a tax for employees to be covered by another source established by government. Also encompassed by the government program would be the unemployed uninsured. When the latter, indirect method of coverage is given to businesses as an option, the plans are known as "play or pay."

Such employer mandate plans represent a middle-of-the-road reform strategy between providing tax subsidies to uninsured individuals, to help them purchase their own private coverage, and a total government takeover of the health care financing system—two other prominent policy positions, associated with Republicans and Democrats, respectively. As such, mandates have been attacked both for proposing too much public intervention and for proposing too little.

From those inclined toward a tax-based solution has come a series of ominous predictions about the economic impact of mandates. By increasing the cost of labor to employers, it is argued, mandates will reduce wages and jobs. Particularly hard hit will be small companies, a sector that accounts for more than half of all working uninsured. Prices of goods and services, too, are expected to rise.

On a more philosophical plane, opponents of mandates question whether guaranteeing universal health care coverage is truly a social responsibility. Or, if granting the point, they maintain that it is unfair to impose this responsibility on private employers. Not entirely consistently, others on the right, including the former Bush administration, have criticized mandates as likely to "cascade into a form of national health insurance" (*The*

219

President's Comprehensive Health Reform Program, 1992)—one scenario is that more and more employers would elect to pay into the publicly operated insurance fund under the play-or-pay option. Another prediction is that a steady aggregation of older and sicker workers drawing on the public fund will lead to unacceptably rising costs for government.

The Working Poor Must Have Coverage

Even outside of the health policy area, experts are arriving at the realization that reforms in many areas of U.S. economic and public policy may hinge on changes that universalize access and bring rising health care costs under some kind of control. . . . And certainly some of the most intractable problems in other areas of social policy, such as welfare reform, depend very much on finding a way to allow the working poor to gain access to health coverage.

Theda Skocpol, *Journal of Health Politics, Policy and Law*, Fall 1993.

Just as many complaints, albeit of a different orientation, come from those who advocate the establishment of a national public health care program in the United States. Some, extrapolating from defects of the current employment-based insurance system, foresee an increasing fragmentation of the insurance market, with private insurance companies calibrating products and prices according to the risk profiles of a greater number of employment groups. Also, the danger of "job lock," wherein people are hesitant to leave a position for one with less generous health benefits, would be worsened if insurers excluded the coverage of preexisting conditions for new group members. [Some] express concern over the special problems this practice would create for women, who are more likely to participate intermittently in the work force. And present experience casts doubt on the ability of multiple separate employers to bargain effectively with insurance companies and health care providers to control rising costs.

In general, critics on the left characterize the employer mandate approach to health care reform as "partial" and "incremental." Their worst fear is not that the adoption of such a strategy will soon lead to national health insurance, but that it will divert needed "comprehensive" and "fundamental" policy change. At last at the point of following the road taken by other Western nations that have confronted similar health system problems, America seems ready to veer off into another historical cul-de-sac. Were a large number of employers to choose to pay into the publicly sponsored insurance plan, proponents of a single national program fear the Medicaid experience writ large—a two-class system of care, which satisfies neither recipients nor providers. . . . Finally, the financing method of an employer mandate is judged regressive in its effects, that is, it inflicts greater burdens on lower-income workers.

These appraisals cast employer mandates as at best ill-considered and at worst a disastrous course of health care reform. To the extent that the brief against mandates has been constructed for political debate, however, it includes the kinds of abstractions, distortions, worst-case scenarios, and straw-man arguments typical in this context. While no analysis can dispel purely ideological preferences for more or less government, careful scrutiny of these various pitfalls can put into perspective the true potential of the mandate strategy. . . .

Who Pays What, When, and How?

One thing is certain. Under all proposed plans the buck stops the same place. Whether it's lost wages, higher prices, higher premiums, or increased taxes, the public will have to foot the bill for expanding health insurance coverage. Within the intricacies of that money trail, however, lie varying equity issues.

Businesses that insure have to pay high premiums because hospital rates are calculated to include uncompensated care of employees of noninsuring businesses. Hence, the charge rings false that to compel noninsuring businesses to offer health benefits is unfair; in this light, it is noninsuring companies that perpetrate inequity, by "free riding" on the cross-subsidies woven into the health care financing system. More and more, business and other group health insurers attempt to resist paying these added costs for hospitals' bad debt and free care—which exceeded $300 million in Massachusetts in fiscal year 1991—by such means as negotiated provider discounts and self-insurance. In 1992 in New Jersey, the courts upheld a related challenge to the state's hospital financing law, which tacks onto the hospital bills of all insured patients (excepting those on Medicare) a 19 percent surcharge to pay for the uninsured. These trends foretell a progressive destabilization of the health care economy and the necessity of bringing all actors into a new systemwide arrangement.

A second frequent equity criticism is that employer mandates penalize struggling small businesses, which are overrepresented among the companies to be affected by new requirements. Current patterns of uninsurance make this problem a real one, although there are several mitigating factors. Any price increases and wage cuts arising from mandates should be felt by all noninsuring small businesses more or less equivalently, maintaining the competitive balance internal to that sector. Also, the leading employer mandate proposals, like Health-

America and the proposal of the National Leadership Coalition for Health Care Reform, contain numerous provisions specifically to soften the impact on small businesses. Included are slower phase-in schedules, small-group insurance reform, special treatment of new businesses, improved tax deductions, and new tax credits for firms with low profit margins. . . .

Finally, there is the question of "regressivity" under employer mandates. The problem is straightforward: assuming some trade-off between new health benefits, payroll taxes, and wages, low-wage earners will be losing a greater proportion of their income. To be sure, a wholly publicly funded program supported by outlays from a progressive income tax would be more egalitarian. However, several points complicate the choice of most suitable funding for health reform.

First, there is the force of tradition to reckon with. The major social insurance entitlements of the American welfare state for unemployment, disability, Medicare, and old-age pensions are all financed primarily by payroll taxes, not general revenues. With government using a sliding-scale fee for enrollees in the publicly sponsored plan and for the premiums of low-income workers in employer plans—a provision of HealthAmerica, for example—an employer mandate would be that much more progressive than these established programs. The opportunity to reduce tax liability by making pretax health plan contributions would be another monetary bonus that mandates would give to those presently working without insurance. Second, although it may be regressive at "take-in," universal health insurance would be progressive at payout to the extent that lower socioeconomic and minority groups have greater need for health services. Third, this awkward combination of regressive and progressive principles, with the regressive dimension outermost, could be critical to avoiding the public perception of universal health care as "welfare." This, in turn, would enhance the initiative's long-term political viability.

Reformers Are Mindful of the Problems

The idea that job lock, more extensive "redlining" of groups and individuals, and other private insurance abuses would worsen under an employer mandate system assumes a half-measure type of reform that is not under serious consideration. Current leading mandate proposals do much more than merely require universal workplace coverage, leaving present market dynamics to shape the outcome. They also embody an array of interventions to remedy the inefficiencies and ineffectiveness of that health care market. Such changes include requirements for communitywide insurance rating and no coverage exclusions on the basis of health status or preexisting conditions. Other pieces of this omnibus overhaul strategy are malpractice reform and administrative and billing simplification. Whether all of these actions will be pursued far enough and buttressed with adequate monitoring is a fair concern. Much of the legislative and administrative process will consist of bargaining with powerful interests over just these issues. Admittedly, this is not a struggle to be taken lightly. But it is simply incorrect at this stage of the national debate to portray mandate reformers as unmindful of such problems. . . .

Employer mandates hold the support of many of the very most powerful actors in the national health policy debate. For example, sponsorship of the HealthAmerica bill, introduced in Congress in July of 1991, came from the Senate Democratic leadership, including Senators Mitchell, Kennedy, Riegle, and Rockefeller. House Ways and Means Chair Dan Rostenkowski's Health Insurance and Cost-Containment Act of 1991 also features a play-or-pay device as its centerpiece. Elsewhere on the political scene, the American Medical Association, for most of the twentieth century this country's most implacable foe of national health plans, has finally cast its vote for reform with an employer mandate strategy. Former presidents Gerald Ford and Jimmy Carter support an employment route to expanded coverage, along with the numerous major business, union, and consumer organizations that came together in the National Leadership Coalition, of which they were honorary cochairs. Some other backers of this general approach—each, of course, with its own preferred variations—include the American Association of Retired Persons, the American Hospital Association, the Pepper Commission, the American Nurses Association, and the AFL-CIO [American Federation of Labor/Congress of Industrial Organizations]. . . .

A predominantly employment-based system is America's indigenous contribution to the international panoply of health insurance approaches. Moreover, of the roughly 35 million Americans who now lack health insurance, 85 percent are workers and their dependents, making the workplace a logical and effective vehicle for addressing the problem of no insurance for the bulk of the population affected. Labor market analysts report a rising trend in businesses' use of part-time and temporary help, "disposable workers," who can be paid lower wages with few fringe benefits. This development makes more comprehensive regulation of privately provided benefit packages not just desirable but an absolute necessity, in order to stem rampant shifting of costs onto private households and government.

Although it is now imperfect, employment-based health insurance nonetheless offers to policymakers a ready-made structure for achieving their objectives of universality and cost constraint. We understand its operational requirements, needed adaptations, and future potential far better than any other model.

*"Employment-related insurance contains built-in
inequities . . . [that] are* endemic *to any
employment-sponsored system."*

Employment-Based
Insurance Is Unjust

Nancy S. Jecker

All employment-based proposals for providing health insurance
are flawed, asserts Nancy S. Jecker in the following viewpoint.
Discrimination of any sort in the workplace spills over into discrimination in providing health care, she declares, using sex-based
bias as an example of this domino effect. Besides, the appropriate
criteria for employment are not directly related to the need for
health care: Those without jobs need insurance more than those
who are employed. Jecker, an associate professor at the University
of Washington School of Medicine, has taught at several institutions specializing in medical ethics and is coauthoring a book, *The
Ends of Medicine: Saying No to Futile Treatment*.

As you read, consider the following questions:

1. Why do working women often receive less insurance
   coverage than men do, according to Jecker?
2. Many women who do not receive employment-related
   insurance are covered by public insurance programs. Why
   does the author maintain that this coverage is unjust?
3. Jecker contends that even forcing all employers to provide
   insurance for all their employees would not solve the
   inequities of employment-based insurance. What points does
   she make to support this?

America's distinctive practice of linking private health insurance to employment is coming under increasing fire. Critics charge that the system produces inequities because it misses so many people. They also fault job-based insurance as inefficient, claiming that it feeds the problem of rising health care costs by distancing consumers from health care costs and thereby encouraging overuse; they argue that employer-based insurance restricts opportunity and lowers productivity because workers feel locked into current jobs for fear of losing benefits. Others worry that employment-sponsored insurance reduces American competitiveness in world markets by raising the cost of American products: in 1990, fully 26 percent of the average company's net earnings went for medical costs.

Since reform of America's health care system is very much on the political agenda today, if employment-based proposals are flawed it is important to state clearly and forcefully why they are. . . . I argue that employment-related insurance contains built-in inequities. Whereas many other objections to employer-sponsored health insurance can be met without abandoning an employer-based framework, the objections I raise are *endemic* to any employment-sponsored system. The objections I put forward constitute an ethical critique of any job-based insurance framework. . . .

Today, workplace health insurance represents the dominant form of private health insurance. . . . [But] even among those who are both employed and insured, health care benefits and access are not uniform. For example, low-wage firms tend to pay a smaller percentage of premium costs and to offer policies with fewer benefits, placing employees at triple jeopardy: they receive less pay, poorer protection, and less tax-exempt employer assistance to defray premium costs. In addition, the federal tax exclusion subsidy is regressive because it offers the most generous after-tax benefits to those with the highest incomes, who would have paid the highest marginal tax rates for their health benefits. [An employer's health insurance contributions can be deducted from company profits like wages, but are not taxable income for employees.] Persons with the lowest incomes, who are in the lower marginal tax brackets, receive the smallest after-tax benefits. . . .

The Domino Effect

To an increasing degree, doubts about the present system raise a more fundamental question: Is America's virtually unique system of linking health insurance to paid labor inherently unjust? Or is it possible to remedy justice problems within the framework of a job-based system? To address such questions, I begin by invoking the familiar idea of a domino effect. . . .

The relevance of the domino effect to health care is straightforward. The distribution of private health insurance is based almost entirely on participation in the paid labor force. If it can be shown that those jobs that provide health insurance are distributed in an unjust way, then tying health insurance to jobs compromises justice in health care. Since the jobs that tend to provide health insurance fall into identifiable categories, we need to examine whether the distribution of these kinds of jobs is just or whether it instead imposes disproportionate burdens on certain groups.

Clearly, there are numerous perspectives from which to evaluate justice in jobs providing health insurance. In making this evaluation, I will focus primarily on inequalities between men and women. The impact of health care financing on men compared with women is a neglected topic but an increasingly important one in light of differences in their socioeconomic status, labor force participation, and health care needs and utilization patterns. Although I use the example of sex-based discrimination, my broader aim is to show that workplace discrimination of any sort, whether based on race, ethnicity, religious affiliation, age, or sexual orientation, creates corresponding injustices in employment-based insurance. . . .

Examining Workplace Discrimination

Although more women today receive health insurance directly from an employer than ever before, employed women are less likely than employed men to receive private health insurance through their job. In 1980, of the 58.4 million men aged fifteen and over who had wage and salary income, 65.4 percent (38.2 million) had an employer or a union that paid all or some of the cost of health insurance; but of the 50.1 million female workers, only 49.7 percent (24.9 million) had an outside contribution. The entire cost of health insurance was paid for 29.6 percent of men but for only 22.9 percent of women.

Working women less often receive private insurance through their employer, first, because eligibility rules continue to reflect a male model of work and male patterns of labor force participation. Full-time, full-year workers more often receive health insurance coverage through the workplace. But, partly as a result of assuming caregiving responsibilities for children and aging relatives, women are more likely to work on a part-time or part-year basis. . . .

Second, working women predominate in nonunion jobs. . . . Not surprisingly, unionized workers generally fare much better with respect to wages and benefits than their nonunionized counterparts, because they have an organized labor force that bargains on their behalf.

A third factor that reduces women's employment-related coverage is that the rate at which women change jobs has greatly increased over the past two decades, while the rate for men has held constant. Partly as a result of child rearing and other caregiving roles, women workers are more likely to enter and leave the work force. They are therefore increasingly vulnerable to clauses in employer insurance plans that exclude or limit coverage for preexisting conditions. . . . The insurance industry uses these clauses to apply higher premiums, waiting periods, condition-specific payment denials, or complete denial of coverage to people with previously existing medical problems. In principle, these clauses are meant to control insurance industry costs by preventing adverse selection—the purchasing of insurance by people who want to pay for insurance only when they need to use it. Yet preexisting condition clauses also block access to care for women and others who participate in the paid labor force intermittently.

Inevitable Injustices

The historical quirk that produced the employer link to and public subsidy of the purchase of health insurance may . . . produce inevitable injustices in the distribution of health insurance. This quirk, on a larger scale, may also be a major contributor to the creation of an unbalanced and ultimately counterproductive distribution of health care resources. Policymakers . . . must consider how to reverse the most damaging aspects of this historic misallocation of resources.

Joan E. Ruttenberg, *Journal of Health Politics, Policy and Law*, Fall 1993.

Fourth, low-paying jobs are less likely to offer health insurance benefits, and women predominate in such jobs. When health insurance premiums rise, many companies with a large proportion of low-wage workers find it increasingly difficult to divert money from wages to health care without reducing wages to unacceptably low levels. As a result, companies such as fast-food restaurants, gasoline stations, and other service jobs keep wages competitive by dropping benefits, including health care. . . .

Public Insurance Is Inadequate

The significance of the sex differential in employer-based insurance lies in the fact that the *public* insurance for which working-age women are eligible is likely to be far less generous than private insurance offered through an employer. Working-age women typically are too young to qualify for Medicare, but often they are not too rich to qualify for Medicaid, the state- and federal-financed health entitlement program for the poor. For every male eighteen years of age and older covered under Medicaid, there are two females aged eighteen and over. But Medicaid is a mixed blessing for women. The health benefits women receive through Medicaid are notoriously meager and inconsistent from one state to the next. Moreover, Medicaid eligibles frequently lack access to mainstream providers, because reimbursement rates are set below costs. Over 25 percent of the nation's privately practicing physicians refuse to treat Medicaid patients; and participation by obstetrician-gynecologists and other key specialists is even lower. . . . Gender inequities will persist so long as public insurance for working-age adults remains inferior to private insurance, and the main route to private insurance continues to be through job categories in which men predominate.

The above discussion reveals quite clearly that women and men do not participate at equal levels in jobs providing health insurance benefits. . . . To the extent that employment disparities between men and women reflect injustice, the link between employment and health insurance merely amplifies this injustice.

The Problem of Dominance

Of course, showing that men are more likely than women to fill jobs that offer health care benefits does not yet establish that such jobs are awarded *unjustly*. Some have argued, to the contrary, that gender differences in employment reflect differences in women's and men's preferences in a free market, rather than invidious discrimination. According to this line of thinking, women voluntarily forgo jobs offering higher salaries and benefits in order to pursue goals outside the paid labor force. . . .

To sidestep this debate, let us suppose for the purposes of argument that jobs providing health insurance coverage are justly distributed among men and women and among all groups in the society. Suppose that such jobs are allocated in conformity with ideal justice standards to which all agree. Would it then be appropriate or desirable to link the distribution of other social goods, such as health care, to the distribution of jobs'?

The strongest argument against linking the distribution of one social good to another involves the problem of dominance. Michael Walzer, who has written extensively in this area, describes dominance as a pattern of distributing diverse goods so that one good, or one set of goods, is determinative of value in all the different spheres of distribution. A good is dominant if the individuals who have it, because they have it, can command a wide range of other goods. For example, wealth and income are the principal dominant goods in our society because they are readily convertible into power, privilege, and position in many areas.

According to Walzer, the need to avoid dominance stems first from the observation that different social goods constitute different distributive spheres in which distinct distributive principles govern. For example, the criteria of intelligence and talent are a fair basis for awarding jobs, but it would be inappropriate to make these the standard for distributing friendship, honor, physical security, food, or shelter. Likewise, something is wrong with the wielding of political power to gain other kinds of benefits, such as superior health care or educational advantages. . . .

Applied to health care, this reasoning suggests that even if jobs are awarded justly, the standards for giving out jobs are not the appropriate standards for apportioning health care. Whereas criteria such as education, work experience, job skills, and freedom from caregiving responsibilities are relevant to evaluating job candidates, these factors should not determine entitlement to health care. Of course, jobs were not made convertible into health care on these grounds. But in hindsight, the de facto effect of an employer-based insurance system has been to make health care available in accordance with the standards used for distributing certain jobs. . . .

The Domino Effect and Dominance

In light of the preceding discussion, one might wonder whether recent proposals to reform America's health care system while retaining a link between jobs and health care can avoid the problems presented here. However, both the domino effect and dominance would persist under mandatory employer health insurance. . . .

Those who favor mandating employer insurance often call attention to its political and strategic advantages. As the vast majority of the uninsured are employed, mandating employer coverage has the distinct advantage of covering the largest subset of the uninsured. In addition, the cost of extended coverage would be borne outside the federal budget and would not appear as a direct tax item. Yet how does mandatory insurance fare in light of the two problems (the domino effect and dominance) discussed above?

By itself, mandatory employer insurance would mean that vastly greater numbers of employees would receive health insurance. Yet eligibility criteria would probably continue to exclude certain categories of workers. For example, the Pepper Commission's Blueprint for Health Care Reform acknowledges that small businesses face significant barriers to voluntary purchasing of health insurance and, for the near future, would seek to reduce barriers while not requiring small businesses to cover their workers. A group calling itself the National Organization of Physicians Who Care proposes achieving mandatory insurance at a reasonable cost through a high deductible, perhaps $1,000. This would continue to place a heavier burden on persons who occupy low-paying jobs. Health Access America, the plan endorsed by the American Medical Association, mandates health insurance only for full-time employees and their families and initially only for large businesses. To the extent that exceptions to categorical coverage are made in job categories that women are more likely than men to fill, inequities between men and women would persist. . . . Even if mandatory employer insurance was supplemented with public insurance for the unemployed, those who rely on a public system would probably continue to receive vastly inferior care. So long as the recipients of public insurance are limited to marginal groups in society, it will remain difficult to maintain an adequate public program. Finally, even assuming that all jobs are *justly* awarded, the unemployed population should not be disqualified from health insurance on the same basis from which it is disqualified from work. Standards that are fair for excluding people from jobs are not necessarily fair for excluding people from health care coverage.

Conclusion

In conclusion, the current system of employer-based health insurance arose through historical events and accidents, rather than through a deliberate and morally thoughtful process. In its wake, patterns of injustice in the distribution of jobs linked to health insurance have compromised justice in health care. . . . Separating health insurance from paid labor force participation may prove a prerequisite to achieving the goal of adequate health care coverage for all.

"Unless we address . . . basic, almost existential questions, we stand little chance of solving our nation's health-care crisis. "

Moral and Ethical Decisions Must Be Made for Regulations to Work

Willard Gaylin

No matter how much fat and waste are cut from the health care system, the country will not be able to provide unlimited health care to everyone who wants it, declares Willard Gaylin in the following viewpoint. Gaylin, a professor of psychiatry at Columbia University Medical School and cofounder and president of The Hastings Center for bioethical research in Briarcliff Manor, New York, maintains that policy debates on resolving the nation's health care crisis have ignored difficult moral and ethical questions that must be faced before sound decisions can be made. Such issues are too important to be left to policymakers, he insists; they must be resolved by open and democratic debate.

As you read, consider the following questions:

1. What "deeper issues of health care" does Gaylin believe should be debated by the public? Why have these issues been ignored, in his view?
2. The author cites an "expanding concept of health" and "the American character" as contributors to an explosion in health care costs. How do these combine, in his opinion, to make the crisis more critical in America than in other countries?

As Hillary Clinton's Task Force on National Health Care Reform completed its deliberations, it sometimes seemed as though the health-care debate we were told the nation was clamoring for had been replaced by a process akin to the selection of a pope. Some five hundred health-care "experts" met behind closed doors over a period of four months, occasionally emitting smoke signals for the media laced with obscure acronyms and buzzwords: HMOs, DRGs, HIPCs (to be pronounced "Hipics," we were instructed), "global budgets," and "managed competition." By now, the public response to the idea of health-care reform is reminiscent of the way most of us feel about our doctors when they begin spouting incomprehensible jargon: we trust that they at least know what they're doing and pray they do no harm.

The most unfortunate thing about this shuttered process is that a remarkable opportunity has been missed. What could have been a wide-open, far-ranging public debate about the deeper issues of health care—our attitudes toward life and death, the goals of medicine, the meaning of "health," suffering versus survival, who shall live and who shall die (and who shall decide)—has been supplanted by relatively narrow quibbles over policy. It is a lot easier and safer for politicians and policymakers to talk about delivery systems, health-product-procurement procedures, and third-party payments than about what care to give a desperately ill child or whether a kidney patient over the age of fifty should be eligible for a transplant. The paradox of our current situation, however, is that unless we address such basic, almost existential questions, we stand little chance of solving our nation's health-care crisis.

Failing to Face the Paradox

Partly because of its unwillingness to confront these issues, the Clinton Administration finds itself tangled in a profound yet largely unacknowledged contradiction. The two key goals of its health-reform plan are (1) to democratize health care—to confront the problem of the 40 million uninsured Americans who can't get adequate care; and (2) to control the ballooning portion of our gross national product that goes to pay for health care. No amount of tinkering with the process of delivery or payment, no number of new tongue-twisting acronyms, can resolve the fundamental contradiction: if you promise everyone access to whatever medical care he or she needs or wants, you will enormously increase the total amount the nation spends on health care—the very costs Clinton was elected to bring under control.

It is of course cost, and not equity, that has driven health care to the fore of the national debate; injustice has never been as urgent a motivating principle as insolvency. The pressure for health-care reform comes on the heels of a staggering surge in spending that threatens to swamp the federal budget and distort our national purposes, not to mention the bottom lines of America's corporations. Twenty-five years ago, 7.6 percent of the gross domestic product was devoted to health, 6.8 percent to education, and 9.7 percent to defense. Today [1993] both defense and education expenditures are roughly 6 percent, whereas health expenditures have climbed to 14 percent of GDP and are likely to reach 18 percent by the end of the decade.

It can easily be argued that it is better to spend money to cure cancer or AIDS than to build more bombs and space stations—and, in fact, that's an argument I agree with. But at the rate by which we are increasing our spending on health care, soon the contest for resources will no longer pit the good guys against the bad guys. For however you define the bad guys, we are quickly running out of them. It is becoming a question of good guys versus good guys, as health-care costs gobble up money that ought to go to those authentic needs that are ancillary, yet essential, to a comprehensive conception of health: such things as drug control, education, crime prevention, housing, and poverty.

What Caused the Explosion in Health-Care Costs?

Most students of the economy, and of the medical economy in particular, agree that the need to contain medical costs is absolute and urgent. The questions that divide us involve how it should be done. And the solutions being offered generally depend on how one accounts for the explosion in health-care costs. Most of the experts and policymakers in Washington have been focusing on the deficiencies and failures of modern medicine: greedy pharmaceutical and insurance companies (not to mention physicians); unnecessary procedures; bureaucratic inefficiency and paperwork; expensive technologies; and so forth. These "efficiency experts," as I call them, have taken control of the debate. . . . They see the solution to our health-care crisis in terms of improving the efficiency of the system. The shibboleths that identify their approach include managed care, HMOs, and managed competition. Implicit in their recommendations is the assumption that the elimination of waste will obviate the need for "rationing" health care.

Opposed to this group are those, myself included, who acknowledge that although there is waste in the system, it is incidental to the basic forces driving up costs. I would argue, in fact, that the greatest part of the increase in health-care costs can best be understood as the result not of the failures of medicine but of its successes. The relentless increase in costs is actually a product of the expanding capabilities of medicine. Implicit in this view is the assumption that controlling waste will save money

233

only in the short haul, and that we had best use the limited time such a strategy will buy to figure out a way to confront the deeper and more challenging reasons for escalating health costs: our unbridled appetite for health care and our continuing expansion of the definition of what constitutes health.

The efficiency experts generally advocate a few basic, businesslike principles that, if adopted, would supposedly solve the cost crisis. The first is the need to reduce the venality of health-care providers, particularly physicians. (If only they had the same generosity of spirit and humanity as other professionals in our society—say, lawyers, accountants, and bankers.) Another way of putting this is that we must cut the fat out of the health-care system. But what system is there that has no fat? Is our goal to make the health-care industry as efficient as the airlines, the automobile industry, the steel industry? Where can we look to find models of efficient managed competition outside of medicine? And where can we look within medicine?

A second bête noire of the efficiency experts is what is called the "halfway technologies"—technologies that extend the life of a patient without actually curing his or her disease. Kidney dialysis is an example. Such technologies sustain people with chronic illnesses at great expense. But the distinction is artificial: since everyone alive is destined to die, *all* medical technologies are halfway technologies. They sustain the human being in the terminal condition we call life.

Preventive Medicine Ultimately Drives Up Costs

This leads directly to the third argument made by the efficiency experts. If only more money were spent on preventive medicine, as opposed to therapeutic medicine, we could solve the problem of health-care costs. The data here are misleading. We all are familiar with the examples: a measles shot costs $8, whereas hospitalization for a child with measles costs $5,000; nine months of prenatal care for a pregnant woman costs $600, whereas medical care for a premature baby for one day costs $2,500. But when you try to extend the economic analysis beyond the individual case to the entire system, it becomes clear that the rationale for preventive medicine is not an economic one. The child who would have died from polio or measles or pertussis will grow up to be a very expensive old man or woman. Preventive medicine drives up the ultimate cost of health care to society by enlarging the population of the elderly and infirm. I am certainly not opposed to preventive medicine, only to irrational arguments for its use. The proper argument for preventive medicine is the grief and misery that it averts and the fact that it allows individuals to lead healthy and productive lives.

The efficiency experts offer several other explanations for ballooning health-care costs, each one based on some others supposed defect in the current system: unnecessary tests, malpractice litigation, bureaucratic waste, profiteering drug companies. Each of these factors adds its penny weight to the scales, but even together they don't begin to account for the sort of quantum leaps in health-care spending we have seen. Even if we were to make angels out of hospital employees and philanthropists out of drug-company executives, we still would not stem the forward march of health-care costs. So what, if not venality and inefficiency, is really driving health costs ever upward into the stratosphere? I would divide the principal causes into four.

Increasing the Number of Sick People

1. The increase in morbidity rates due to good medicine. It is often difficult for laypeople to appreciate that good medicine does not reduce the percentage of people with illnesses in our population (what is called the morbidity rate); it *increases* that percentage. There are more people wandering the streets of the cities of the United States with arteriosclerotic heart disease, diabetes, essential hypertension, and other expensive chronic diseases than there are in Iraq, Nigeria, or Colombia. Good medicine keeps *sick* people alive, thereby increasing the number of sick people in the population; patients who are killed by their disease are no longer a part of the population. Even outright cures of diseases ultimately add to medical costs. We no longer talk about diphtheria rates or whooping-cough rates, even though those were the two leading causes of death in children for many generations. Those diseases have ceased to exist. But they were rarely expensive. The child either lived or died, and, for the most part, did so quickly and cheaply.

2. The expanding concept of health. Health today does not mean what it did a hundred years ago. If I might begin by casting stones at my own glass house, consider the case of psychiatry, though psychiatry is not the worst offender. The fact is that the patients I deal with in my daily practice would not have been considered mentally ill in the nineteenth century. Mental illness then was rigidly defined. Those considered mentally ill were insane—patently different from you and me—and they were put into hospitals. The leading causes of mental illness were tertiary syphilis and schizophrenia. This, more or less, was psychiatry (a minor branch of neurology) at the turn of the century, before the arrival of its genius, Sigmund Freud. Freud decided that people did not have to be exclusively either crazy or sane, but that a normal person, like himself or people he knew, could be partly crazy. These "normal" people, who were still in touch with reality, exhibited only isolated symptoms of irrationality—phobias, compulsions, etc. Freud invented a new category of mental diseases now called "neuroses," thereby vastly increasing the population of the mentally ill.

Some thirty years later, Wilhelm Reich decided that one does not even have to display mental symptoms to be mentally ill, that one can suffer from "character disorders." The personalities of even completely asymptomatic individuals might so limit their productivity or pleasure in life that we are justified in diagnosing them as mentally ill.

Then medicine "discovered" the psychosomatic disorders. There are people with no symptoms of mental illness who have *physical* conditions with psychic roots—peptic ulcers, ulcerative colitis, migraine headache, allergies, and the like. These people, too, were now classified as mentally ill. By such sophisticated expansion of the category, we eventually managed to get some 60 percent to 70 percent (as one serious study found) of the residents of the Upper East Side of Manhattan into the population of the mentally ill.

"Discovering" New Diseases

What has happened in mental health has happened across the board in medicine: we have radically altered our concept of what it means to be sick or healthy. Probably the best way to understand this process is to consider how medicine goes about "discovering" new diseases.

Most people assume that medical researchers first uncover an illness and then seek a cure for it. This, of course, does happen; the infectious diseases are the paradigm case. What is less familiar, but is becoming more common, is the opposite mechanism: we discover a cure and then invent a disease to go with it.

As I am writing this article I am using reading glasses. These reading glasses are paid for by a health insurer, based on the diagnosis of "presbyopia" (an eye "disease") made by an ophthalmologist (a specialty physician). Before the invention of the lens there was no such disease as presbyopia; there were also no ophthalmologists. Old people weren't expected to read. A decline in faculties was simply part of the aging process; with age, sight would be impaired or lost, as would be hearing, potency, and fertility. As we began to find treatments to delay the aging processes, we reclassified various aspects of aging as "diseases."

This vast expansion of the concept of health can be demonstrated in surgery, orthopedics, gynecology—indeed, in any field of medicine. Infertility, for example, was not considered a disease until this generation; before then, it was simply a God-given condition. With the advances of modern medicine—including artificial insemination, in vitro fertilization, and surrogate mothering—new cures were discovered for "illnesses" that now had to be invented. All of them make demands on the health-care dollar. Another example: People do not get their knees or elbows operated on merely to continue to function or be employable; most of us do not work at jobs requiring physical strength. Many operations on the knee are performed strictly so that the patient can continue to play golf or ski; it is the same with elbow operations. Are these justifiable "medical" expenses? If one is free of pain except on the tennis court, is one "ill"? Should "inability to play tennis" be classified as an insurable disease?

Life-and-Death Decisions

3. The seduction of technology and the deception of marketplace models. All of us know about how doctors can be seduced by medical technology—how, for example, the ubiquity of delivery-room fetal monitors (which alert obstetricians to the merest hint of fetal distress) has contributed to a surge in cesarean sections. But it is not only the physician who is seduced by technology; the patient and her family are, too—and not because of an infatuation with gadgetry, but because of the nature of decision-making in matters of life and death. Decision-making becomes distorted whenever extreme risks are involved; also, our perceptions of probability vary significantly depending on the setting.

A driver is probably safer in an $80,000 Mercedes than in an $8,000 Isuzu, but few people are likely to mortgage the house for the Mercedes, at least not for reasons of safety. Similarly, driving 65 miles an hour carries a greater risk of a fatal accident than driving 55, yet this well-publicized fact doesn't seem to keep many drivers under the speed limit. The possible consequence is too remote; on a drive to Cape Cod one is thinking about a dip in the ocean, not the imminence of death. But these perceptions change in a hospital setting. Imagine if a doctor were to tell a patient that he sees no sign of a tumor in the X ray and that though a CAT scan *might* pick up the 1 percent of tumors that X rays miss, he is not sure it is worth the extra money. The patient would fire him on the spot. He wants any edge, however minute, when what is at stake is the life of his child, his wife, or himself. When the doctor then tells him, after a negative CAT scan, that an MRI might still pick up a tumor, the patient demands the MRI. He will mortgage the house for that, although the statistical validity of doing so, compared with exercising prudence on the highway, may make no sense. Death has a greater reality in the hospital setting. People will pay anything to defend against the possibility of death, all the more so when the money involved doesn't come directly out of their own pockets.

Because our approach to medical technology is special, we are wrong to assume that the marketplace in medical technology will ever follow classical patterns. Generally, as technologies mature and become more prevalent their costs decline rapidly. I remember once discussing with a brilliant money manager the perilous rise in the cost of medicine. I was being unduly pessimistic, he claimed—it is in the nature of new technologies to become cheaper over time, and he cited the ballpoint pen, the CD player, and the computer as examples. What he failed to realize is that highly specialized technologies controlled by small groups of manufacturers do not respond to the marketplace in the same way that mass-produced items do. Nor did he take into account the fact that, in health matters, people are willing to pay substantially more money for relatively minor improvements. When what is being improved is life expectancy rather than, say, the fidelity of sound coming off of a recording, all the rules change. Medical technology will continue to be expensive simply because it pays to market a 1 percent improvement even though it might be 100 percent more expensive. Armed with this knowledge, a manufacturer will rush to market with an expensive procedure or a drug only marginally superior to one that is already available at a significantly lower price.

Facing Up to Divisive Moral Issues

We might be better off if we face up to the major political and moral issues that divide us. One way to do that would be to experiment a bit more with what I call "moral federalism." Both sides in our moral debates want to universalize their positions: Condoms should be distributed to teenagers in *every* school or they should be distributed in *none*. In reality, different localities and different states will try different approaches, and this is how it should be. . . . A policy of encouraging particular rather than universal moralities may violate consistency and philosophical principles, but it makes a good deal of political sense. Eventually, universal moral principles may emerge as people learn that their particular moralities are, when actually implemented, more problematic than they had assumed.

Alan Wolfe, *The Wilson Quarterly*, Summer 1993.

---

4. The American character and appetite. People often ask how nations such as England and Canada can provide health care comparable to ours for much less money. First of all, they use a single-party payment system—that is, the government pays everyone's health-care costs directly, an option, though highly efficient, that we seem unwilling even to consider. Second, they are not, in fact, offering comparable services. Their health-care system does not make nearly as much use of technology, and they are willing, at least for now, to settle for less. (But this appears to be changing: most nations with managed care are now accelerating their health-care spending at a *more* rapid rate than we are.)

The Nature of the American Character

The health-care crisis is at its most critical in America not only because we are the preeminent high-technology culture but also because of the nature of the American character. I was reminded of this during a seminar at which a distinguished English Marxist was holding forth on the venality of the American medical system by citing the higher rates of hernia-repair surgery done in America as compared with England. Since the incidence of hernias is the same in both countries, he interpreted the increased rate of repairs as the product of unnecessary surgery, driven by American greed. It occurred to me that there might be at least two or three other explanations. The simplest, of course, and the one that turns out to be the most accurate, is the funnel effect. Under the medical system in England, health-care services are free and widely distributed. But in order to control costs, and also to save hospital space, voluntary surgery to correct conditions that are not life-threatening is limited to a relatively small number of hospital beds. This results in a long waiting period—a six-lane highway leading to a single tollbooth will allow fewer cars through in an hour than one with six tollbooths. Limited facilities simply mean that the system allows for fewer hernias to be repaired in a given period of time. The disparity does not require the greed of the American surgeon.

The deeper explanation, however, is rooted in differences between the American and the British characters. Americans want things solved completely and they want them solved now; they don't want to hear about restrictions, especially on something like health care. I can easily conceive of a typical midland Englishman actually *preferring* to walk around wearing a truss, reflexively moving his hands to his lower abdomen every time he coughs, rather than rushing off for surgery to repair his hernia.

The American character *is* different. Perhaps because of our frontier heritage, Americans refuse to believe there are limits—even to life itself. Consider the struggle in America to define such terms as "death with dignity," which really means death without dying, and "growing old gracefully," a related term that, on closer analysis, means living a long time without aging. Dying in one's sleep at ninety-two after having won three sets of tennis from one's forty-year-old grandson that afternoon and having made love to one's wife twice that same evening— this is about the only scenario I have found most American men will accept as fulfilling their idea of death with dignity and growing old gracefully.

Medical costs will bankrupt this country if they continue on their current trajectory. And there are no data to demonstrate that improved management techniques will solve the problem. "Managed care" and "managed competition" might save money in the short run (though the examples of some other managed industries—such as the utilities and airlines—do not inspire confidence). But the bulk of the savings achieved by Health Maintenance Organizations has been achieved by cutting back on expensive, unprofitable facilities such as burn centers, neonatal-intensive-care units, emergency rooms, and the like. In other words, HMOs conduct what amounts to a hidden form of health-care rationing—confident in the knowledge that municipal and university hospitals are still around to pick up the slack.

As the managers of HMOs know only too well, the surest ways to contain health-care spending are to limit access to health care and to rethink our ever-expanding concept of health. But if we must have allocation, the process should not be hidden from public view or determined by a small group of health-care professionals. It requires open discussion and wide participation. When what we are rationing is life itself, the decisions must be subjected to public scrutiny and debate. The first step is to admit to the cruel necessity of rationing health care. The second is to set limits on health care according to principles of equity and justice.

The kinds of questions we will need to debate can be divided into three: issues of access (how do we decide who gets to receive a scarce health resource?), egress (how long may they receive it?), and allocation (what medical services can the system as a whole provide to everyone?).

Debating the Real Questions

1. Access. We can no longer leave to the marketplace decisions about access to medical care. We do not want kidneys to be sold to the highest bidder, and yet we now tolerate something perilously close to that. People can still use influence, power, position, and simply money to buy access to lifesustaining services. It is disgraceful to see a parent forced to "advertise" for a liver for her baby on *Oprah* while the governor of Pennsylvania is rushed to the head of the line for his heart and liver transplant. Access to scarce health resources must be organized on some equitable basis—even if equitable does not necessarily mean full coverage for everybody for everything.

There are various factors we might consider in evaluating competing claims on scarce and expensive services. One obvious consideration is age. Most of us would agree that a seventy-two-year-old man, let alone a ninety-two-year-old man, has less of a claim on an organ transplant than a thirty-two-year-old mother or a sixteen-year-old boy, all other things being equal. And yet proponents of such policies are commonly attacked as "ageists."

These are never easy decisions. They force us to face our own mortality and demand that we look beyond our own sympathies and interests. But they must be confronted nevertheless. When I recently presented the problem of access to an interdisciplinary class of law, medical, and theology students, the students' first response was that a lottery would be the best way to guarantee fairness. Yet leaving such an important decision to a lottery—precisely because it seeks to avoid questions of justice and fairness—is itself immoral. If my name were put into a drawing for access to a lifesaving resource along with my daughter's or my granddaughter's, and my name were the lucky one drawn, my first act upon recovery would be to throttle the idiot who set up such a system. Claims on life must be based on enunciated values. Only after we have decided on our priorities and established our categories should we consider using a lottery, as we have done when we have operated a wartime draft.

When Should Access End?

2. *Egress.* The ethical dilemmas do not end with decisions about access to scarce services or technologies; now comes the even trickier (and seldom asked) question of deciding if and when that access should end. Imagine a system in which we have a limited number of artificial-heart devices. We must allocate not only a patient's access but also the amount of time he or she may have on this lifesaving machine. A year might seem insufficient; so might five. But forever until death? Even when someone else, much younger, will be dying while waiting for access to that very machine? So perhaps we pull the plug after an agreed-upon period—say, ten years, or twenty. Now we have been forced out onto the treacherous moral ground of euthanasia—and yet this is precisely where our technology, coupled with our funding crisis, is taking us.

It is ludicrous to think we can take away a lifesaving technology once we have introduced it. Since every new medical technology, however expensive, quickly becomes part of the therapeutic norm (and, from the patients' point of view, no longer a privilege but a right), we might be better off deciding in advance not to develop certain new technologies. Such an argument is now being made by bioethicists in debates over the boundaries of future medical research. Some argue, for example, that in view of the health-care system's current economic problems, we ought not develop a left-ventricular pump (essentially, a portable artificial heart). But how can we limit scientific inquiry? We can't—but we can debate what we as a society are willing to fund, just as we now debate whether we really need a supercollider.

3. *Allocation.* What medical services can our society afford to provide to everyone? Here lies the political mine field that the Clinton Administration has apparently decided not to cross. From all indications, the Clinton plan will offer a very generous package of "basic" health-care benefits to be made available to everyone. Guided by a group of "policy wonks" and quants disdainful of the sticky dilemmas inherent in moral reasoning and terrified by the ambiguities inevitable when dealing with values, the Clinton task force has indulged in the wishful thinking that we *can* have it all—as long as we get the flow charts and systems theory right. By focusing exclusively on cost efficiency, the Clinton plan will do little to disturb the self-deceptive and self-destructive belief that we can meet every American's every "health" need: artificial organs, genetic screening, transplants, unproven AIDS drugs, psychotherapy for unhappiness, surgery for the tennis elbow, intensive care for the infirm elderly as well as for the two-pound fetus.

Tragic Choices Must Be Made

But we cannot do everything for everybody. Limited resources will force us to make tragic choices among competing health needs—if not now, under the Clinton plan, then very soon. To the uninitiated, these may look like medical choices, best made by medical professionals. In fact, they are not medical choices; they are moral and ethical ones, best made by all of us, struggling toward consensus through the usual, sloppy devices of democratic government.

Perhaps this is too much to ask of a governmental task force. But there is a precedent for just such a public process. Five years ago the state of Oregon attempted to confront the very dilemma the Clinton task force has chosen to duck. Oregon sought to guarantee a basic health-care package to everyone; at the same time, it acknowledged that doing so would bankrupt the state unless some hard choices were made about what should constitute "basic health care." Not all health services could be included. In other words, Oregon faced up to the issue of allocation, and it did so out in the open: in a series of town meetings and a statewide "health parliament," issues of access and medical priorities were debated publicly, sometimes fiercely. The state's health commission then published a comprehensive list of medical conditions and treatments, each ranked according to its costs and benefits. More debate ensued; the list was revised. Finally, the legislature decided exactly where on the revised list the state could afford to draw the necessary cutoff line: it would pay for hip replacements and neonatal care, for example, but not liver transplants or in vitro fertil-

242

ization. (Oregonians who still wanted such treatments were free to pay for them.) By conducting much of this process in public, the health commission was able to develop a consensus behind some otherwise unpopular decisions.

The Oregon plan is by no means perfect. But at least the state has addressed the uncomfortable truth that they cannot have equity in their health-care system without making anguished, even tragic choices. Even more important, the people of Oregon have had a searching public conversation about new technologies and medical priorities, chronic care and cosmetic surgery—about how much health care they can afford and what it really means to be healthy. That is probably a lot more than the rest of us can expect from the narrow, numbing discussion of systems and policies and acronyms that the President insists on calling a health-care debate.

Periodical Bibliography

The following articles have been selected to supplement the diverse views presented in this chapter.

Susan Hershberg Adelman	"Tort Reform Must Be Part of Health Care Reform," *American Medical News*, April 12, 1993. Available from 515 N. State St., Chicago, IL 60610.
Doug Bandow	"Health Care Reform: A Placebo May Be the Best Remedy," *Business & Society Review*, Summer 1993. Available from 200 W. 57th St., New York, NY 10019.
Peter J. Ferrara	"Managed Competition: Less Choice and Competition, More Costs and Government in Health Care," *The Heritage Foundation Backgrounder*, June 29, 1993. Available from 214 Massachusetts Ave. NE, Washington, DC 20002-4999.
Peter Kerr	"Insurers Fear They'd Be the Big Losers in a World of Managed Health Care," *The New York Times*, October 1, 1993.
Susan Moran	"Regulation: Bad Medicine for Doctors," *Insight*, September 27, 1993.
Robert Pear	"Medical Malpractice Study Finds Unjust Payments Are Rare," *The New York Times*, November 1, 1992.
Janice Perrone	"Physician, Police Thyself: Can Renewed Emphasis on Ethics Blunt Government Regulation?" *American Medical News*, April 27, 1992.
Raymond Scalettar	"Dear Congress: An MD's Letter from the Front," *American Medical News*, May 24, 1993.
Michael S. Sparer	"States and the Health Care Crisis," *Journal of Health Politics, Policy, and Law*, Vol. 18, No. 2, Summer 1993. Available from Duke University Press, 6697 College Station, Durham, NC 27708.
P. Roy Vagelos	"Healthcare Reform: Supporting America's Vision," *Vital Speeches of the Day*, December 15, 1992.
Michael Waldholz	"Drug Makers' Image Ills Are Self-Induced," *The Wall Street Journal*, March 30, 1993.

Glossary

acupuncture   The Chinese practice of puncturing the body with needles at specific points to ease pain or cure disease.

AMA   American Medical Association; the largest and most influential professional association for physicians in the United States.

chiropractic medicine   A type of medical practice in which the spine and other body parts are manipulated and adjusted to ease pain and cure disease.

D.C.   Doctor of chiropractic.

defensive medicine   Medical practice in which physicians order an excessive number of medical tests and procedures or perform unnecessary surgeries to protect themselves from malpractice lawsuits.

FDA   Food and Drug Administration; the federal agency charged with protecting public health by ensuring that foods, cosmetics, and medicines are safe, effective, and honestly labeled.

GNP   gross national product; a nation's total output of goods and services in a given period, usually one year.

HMO   health maintenance organization; a type of prepaid medical service in which members pay a monthly or yearly fee for all health care, including hospitalization. Most HMOs are staffed by physicians who are members of medical groups. Because costs to patients are fixed, preventive medicine is stressed to avoid costly hospitalization.

holistic medicine   A type of medical practice that stresses taking into account a patient's mental, emotional, and spiritual concerns as well as his or her physical symptoms of disease.

homeopathy   A system of therapy based on the theory that certain substances that normally cause disease conditions will, when administered in extremely minute amounts, instead help rid the body of those same conditions.

managed care   A method of delivering and monitoring health care, often through the use of HMOs; under a managed-care system, each individual is assigned a primary-care physician who acts as the "gatekeeper" of medical care—providing individuals with most of their medical care and prescribing special treatments and referrals when needed. The purpose of managed care is to contain health care costs while ensuring access to quality care.

managed competition   A health care policy that combines free-market forces with government regulation, as a way of providing high-quality care at the lowest cost; large groups of businesses and individuals would join together to purchase health care, and networks of insurance companies and health providers would compete for their business.

NCHS   National Center for Health Statistics; the federal agency that collects statistics concerning Americans' health.

245

NHP   National Health Program; the Canadian health care system.

NIH   National Institutes of Health; the federal agency that conducts and supports biomedical research into the cause, cure, and prevention of disease.

osteopathy   A medical practice based on the theory that most ailments are caused by the misalignment of bones and muscles and can be treated by manipulating these body parts. Such treatment is often supplemented with drugs and, if needed, surgery.

PAC   political action committee; an organization formed by a corporation, labor union, or association to raise money for political activity.

pay or play   A system of providing medical care supported by employer contributions; under a pay-or-play system, an employer must choose either to provide health insurance for its employees ("play") or to contribute to a government-administered fund to provide health insurance for all who are not covered by their employers ("pay").

PPO   preferred provider organization; a managed-care arrangement in which doctors contract individually with a health plan, agreeing to provide medical care for fixed fees.

primary care   Medical care that provides preventive services and treats minor illnesses; practiced mainly by family physicians, pediatricians, and internists.

rationing   The practice of controlling the amount of a certain commodity, such as health care, that individuals can acquire; rationing health care would mean that the use of certain expensive medical procedures would be controlled so that not everyone who desires the procedure would be able to receive it.

single-payer   A health plan in which one organization, usually the federal or state government, would pay for all health care, eliminating the need for third-party payers such as insurance companies.

For Further Discussion

Chapter 1

1. Advances in medicine have saved the lives of millions of Americans in recent decades. Yet William B. Schwartz blames these very advances for rising health care costs. Do you think, as Schwartz does, that expensive medical procedures should be rationed? Defend your answer.

2. Bryce J. Christensen cites the decline of the traditional family as one cause of America's health care crisis. What points in his argument are persuasive? What points seem less convincing?

3. Most of the contributors to this chapter point to specific causes of the health care crisis and offer specific solutions. How does Nathan Karp's view differ from those of the other authors? How does Fred Barnes's view differ from those of the other authors? Are their views convincing? Why or why not?

Chapter 2

1. Why does Arnold S. Relman believe physicians share in the blame for the health care crisis? From your personal experience with your physician, do you agree with his assessment? Explain your answer, perhaps by describing positive or negative experiences you have had with your physician.

2. Steven A. Schroeder is a general physician. Joseph D. Wassersug is a retired heart and lung specialist. How do you think their occupations affect their views concerning the balance of general physicians to specialists? What convincing points do the authors make in support of their views?

3. Mike Royko defends the high salaries physicians receive. What facts does he cite to support his opinion? Think about the training and expense physicians go through to practice their profession and the time and talent required of them. Then think about the high salaries, the high status, and the other benefits of being a physician. Do you think physicians deserve the pay and respect they receive? Defend your answer.

4. Throughout his viewpoint, Charles B. Inlander compares physicians to greedy vultures. How does this comparison af-

fect your own opinion? Is Inlander persuasive? Would he be more persuasive or less persuasive if he used a less dramatic method of conveying his opinion? Explain your answer.

Chapter 3

1. Sara Solovitch, Carolyn Copeland, and George Magner all base their opinions about alternative medicine on their personal experiences. Do you find their viewpoints persuasive? Why or why not? Are such personal accounts more or less effective than opinions based on facts such as statistics or opinion polls? Explain your answer.

2. Why does James S. Gordon believe physicians are partly to blame for Americans' increased interest in alternative medicine? How does Stephen Barrett counter such arguments? Which author is more persuasive? Using information from the chapter and from your own experiences, discuss why Americans are increasingly turning to alternative medicine.

3. Stephen J. Press is founder and president of the International Federation of Sports Chiropractic. George Magner says he was injured by a chiropractic treatment. How do these facts affect the persuasiveness of their viewpoints? What experiences, if any, have you or people you know had with chiropractic medicine?

Chapter 4

1. In some nations, the government pays for all of the citizens' health care needs. Steffie Woolhandler and David U. Himmelstein, who support such a system, refer to it as "nationalized health care." Jarret B. Wollstein, who opposes it, calls the system "socialized medicine." Why do you think Wollstein chooses to use the word "socialized"? What implications might some people associate with this word? How might these implications affect their perceptions of government-run health care?

2. Alain C. Enthoven supports managed competition as the solution to America's health care crisis. Enthoven helped originate the idea of managed competition. How does this fact affect your opinion of his viewpoint? What would be the benefits of managed competition, according to Enthoven? How does Judith Randal counter arguments for managed competition?

3. Nat Hentoff is a well-known columnist respected by many for his advocacy of individual rights. Daniel Callahan is a well-known medical ethicist respected by many for his insightful opinions concerning complex medical issues. Compare Hentoff's and Callahan's views concerning health care rationing. Why do you think the issue of rationing is such a sensitive, emotional one? What are some other issues that divide intelligent, thoughtful, ethical people into opposite sides?

4. Elaine Bernard advocates the U.S. adoption of a health care system similar to Canada's. Edmund F. Haislmaier opposes such a system. What are the positive aspects of Canada's system? What problems does it face? From what you have read, does it seem to you that Canadians are well served by their health care system? Why or why not? Do you think the United States should adopt a Canadian-style system? Why or why not?

Chapter 5

1. Jose Lozano is a physician and Philip H. Corboy is an attorney who represents victims of medical malpractice. How do you think their professions affect their opinions concerning malpractice awards? Do they give their arguments more credibility or less? Why?

2. Jose Lozano and many other physicians argue that their malpractice premiums are too high and that the malpractice system unfairly punishes physicians for their mistakes. Philip H. Corboy and others argue in turn that the malpractice system is the only way patients can be repaid for injuries they suffer because of physicians' incompetence. Who do you think has the best argument? Explain your answer. Discuss ways to improve the system so that it (a) disciplines incompetent physicians; (b) protects competent physicians from excessive premiums; and (c) helps victims of medical malpractice.

3. How does Murray Weidenbaum defend the high prices pharmaceutical companies charge for prescription drugs? Why does Lionel Van Deerlin believe these high prices are indefensible? Which author is more persuasive? Why?

Organizations to Contact

The editors have compiled the following list of organizations concerned with the issues debated in this book. The descriptions are derived from materials provided by the organizations. All have publications or information available for interested readers. The list was compiled on the date of publication of the present volume; names, addresses, and phone numbers may change. Be aware that many organizations take several weeks or longer to respond to inquiries, so allow as much time as possible. Note that there are thousands of health care organizations in the United States; this is just a small sampling. For more information, consult reference sources such as the *Encyclopedia of Associations*.

American Academy of Family Physicians
8880 Ward Pkwy.
Kansas City, MO 64114
(816) 333-9700
fax: (816) 822-0580

The academy is the professional association of family physicians. It works to serve family physicians and to increase the public's understanding of the profession. The academy publishes the monthly *AAFP Reporter*, a newsletter covering socioeconomic issues and legislative news affecting medicine; a triennial directory; and the monthly *American Family Physician*.

American Chiropractic Association
1701 Clarendon Blvd.
Arlington, VA 2229
(703) 276-8800
fax: (703) 243-2593

The association works to promote chiropractic medicine and to serve chiropractors. It supports legislation that increases the use of chiropractic medicine, and expands the public's knowledge concerning the profession. The association conducts studies and maintains a library. It publishes the monthly newsletter *ACA/FYI*, an annual directory, and the monthly *Journal of Chiropractic*.

American Holistic Medical Association
4101 Lake Boone Trail, Suite 201
Raleigh, NC 27607
(919) 787-5146
fax: (919) 787-4916

The association includes medical doctors, osteopaths, and others interested in practicing, using, and promoting holistic medicine. It provides the public with referrals to holistic physicians. Its publications include the bimonthly magazine *Holistic Medicine*, the books *Fitness Guidelines* and *Nutritional Guidelines*, and various brochures.

American Medical Association (AMA)
515 N. State St.
Chicago, IL 60610
(312) 464-4818
fax: (312) 464-4184

The AMA is the primary professional association of physicians in the United States. Founded in 1847, it disseminates information to its members and the public concerning medical breakthroughs, medical and health legislation, educational standards for physicians, and other issues concerning medicine and health care. The AMA operates a library and offers many publications, including the weekly *Journal of the American Medical Association*, the weekly newspaper *American Medical News*, and journals covering specific types of medical specialties.

American Public Health Association (APHA)
1015 15th St. NW
Washington, DC 20005
(202) 789-5600
fax: (202) 789-5681

The American Public Health Association comprises health professionals and others interested in protecting and promoting personal, mental, and environmental health. It researches public health issues, sponsors a job placement service for health professionals, and works to educate the public concerning health matters. In addition to books, manuals, and pamphlets, the association's publications service offers the *American Journal of Public Health* monthly and *The Nation's Health* ten times a year. *The Nation's Health* reports on current and proposed legislation, regulations, and policy issues affecting public health.

American Society of Law and Medicine
765 Commonwealth Ave., 16th Fl.
Boston, MA 02215
(617) 262-4990
fax: (617) 437-7596

The society's members include physicians, attorneys, health care administrators, and others interested in the relationship between law and medicine and in health law. The organization has an information clearinghouse and a library. It publishes the quarterlies *American Journal of Law and Medicine* and *Law, Medicine, and Health Care*, the periodic *ASLM Briefings*, and books such as *Legal and Ethical Aspects of Health Care for the Elderly* and *Health Care Labor Law*.

Health Insurance Association of America (HIAA)
1025 Connecticut Ave. NW
Washington, DC 20036
(202) 223-7780

HIAA is the primary lobby of accident and health insurance firms. It provides the public with information on the need for insurance and promotes legislation that furthers the interests of the insurance industry. The association has many publications, including consumer guides to health insurance programs; the periodic *Medical Practice Assessment Report* and *Research Bulletin*; and the annual *Sourcebook of Health Insurance Data*.

Health Policy Advisory Center (Health/PAC)
47 W. 14th St., No. 300
New York, NY 10011
(212) 627-1847

The goal of Health/PAC is to monitor the health care system for those consumers, health care workers, and others who wish to provide low-cost, high-quality health care for all. The center believes that the health care system should encourage the prevention of illness and should not simply serve the needs of the health care industry. It publishes the *Health/PAC Bulletin* quarterly and offers special reports, pamphlets, books, and educational materials.

The Heritage Foundation
214 Massachusetts Ave. NE
Washington, DC 20002
(202) 546-4400

The Heritage Foundation is a public-policy research institute that supports limited government and the free-market system. It opposes nationalized health care and has proposed its own health care reform plan that minimizes government involvement. The foundation publishes the quarterly journal *Policy Review* as well as monographs, books, and papers concerning health care in America.

International Health Policy and Management Institute
c/o Paul Detrick
10133 Dunn Rd., Suite 400
St. Louis, MO 63136
(314) 355-0095

The institute, whose members include health policymakers, hospital administrators, physicians, business leaders, and educators, is dedicated to improving the public's knowledge of health care economics. Its goals are to improve the financing and delivery of health care and to encourage research into health policy issues. The institute publishes research reports, books, monographs, and the quarterly newsletter *International Perspectives*.

National Association of Managed Care Physicians
Innsbrook Corporate Center
5040 Sadler Rd., Suite 103
Glen Allen, VA 23060-6124
(800) 722-0376
fax: (804) 747-5316

The association includes physicians and other health care professionals who work in managed-care programs, such as health maintenance organizations. It aims to help those who work in managed-care programs and to ensure that patients in such programs receive quality care. The association monitors legislative issues and lobbies for legislation that benefits managed-care physicians. It offers seminars, educational programs, research programs, a speakers bureau, placement services, and an informational clearinghouse. Its publications include the quarterly *NAMCP News* and the monograph series *NAMCP Guide to Managed Care.*

National Center of Employers on Health Care Action
240 Crandon Blvd., Suite 110
PO Box 220
Key Biscayne, FL 33149
(305) 361-2810
fax: (305) 361-2842

The center aims to educate and assist employers in providing cost-effective, high-quality health care programs for their employees. It conducts research and provides information on health care management and lobbies the U.S. Congress concerning health legislation affecting employers. It publishes the *Employers' Guide to Purchasing Managed Health Care Services* periodically, the *Health Action Newsletter* monthly, and two directories on health maintenance organizations and preferred-provider organizations.

National Committee for Quality Health Care
1500 K St. NW, Suite 360
Washington, DC 20005
(202) 347-5731
fax: (202) 347-5836

The committee includes a wide variety of professionals and organizations involved in the health care industry. Its goal is to improve the quality of health care in the United States. It publishes the *Quality Bulletin* and *Quality Outlook* six times a year, pamphlets, reports, and the books *Critical Condition: America's Health Care in Jeopardy* and *An American Health Strategy: Ensuring the Availability of Quality Health Care.*

National Council Against Health Fraud (NCAHF)
PO Box 1276
Loma Linda, CA 92354-1276
(909) 824-4690
fax: (909) 824-4838

The NCAHF is a voluntary health organization that focuses on health misinformation, fraud, and quackery as public health problems. It offers a resource list of more than six hundred articles concerning health fraud and publishes the bimonthly *Bulletin Board,* a bimonthly newsletter, books, and book list.

Bibliography of Books

Henry J. Aaron	*Serious and Unstable Condition: Financing America's Health Care.* Washington, DC: The Brookings Institution, 1991.
Lu Ann Aday	*At Risk in America: The Health and Health Care Needs of Vulnerable Populations in the United States.* San Francisco: Jossey-Bass, 1993.
George J. Annas	*The Rights of Patients.* Totowa, NJ: Humana Press, 1992.
David Aquilina et al.	*Driving Down Health-Care Costs: Strategies and Solutions.* New York: Panel Publications, Inc., 1992.
Joseph L. Bast, Richard C. Rue, and Stuart A. Wesbury Jr.	*Why We Spend Too Much on Health Care.* Chicago: The Heartland Institute, 1992.
Lisa Belkin	*First, Do No Harm.* New York: Simon & Schuster, 1993.
Arnold Bennett and Orvill Adams, eds.	*Looking North for Health: What We Can Learn From Canada's Health Care System.* San Francisco: Jossey-Bass, 1993.
Robert J. Blendon and Tracy Stelzer Hyams, eds.	*Reforming the System: Containing Health Care Costs in an Era of Universal Coverage.* Washington, DC: Faulkner & Gray's Healthcare Information Center, 1992.
Thomas J. Bole III and William B. Bondeson	*Rights to Health Care.* Dordrecht, Netherlands: Academic Publishers, 1991.
Troyen Brennan	*Just Doctoring.* Berkeley: University of California Press, 1991.
Howard Brody	*The Healer's Power.* New Haven: Yale University Press, 1992.
Kurt Butler	*A Consumer's Guide to "Alternative Medicine": A Close Look at Homeopathy, Acupuncture, Faith Healing, and Other Unconventional Treatments.* Buffalo: Prometheus Books, 1992.
Stuart M. Butler and Edmund F. Haislmaier, eds.	*A National Health System for America.* Washington, DC: The Heritage Foundation, 1989.
Kevin M. Cahill	*Imminent Peril: Public Health in a Declining Economy.* New York: The Twentieth Century Fund Press, 1991.

Arthur L. Caplan — *If I Were a Rich Man Could I Buy a Pancreas?: And Other Essays on the Ethics of Health Care.* Bloomington and Indianapolis: Indiana University Press, 1992.

Harris Dienstfrey — *Where the Mind Meets the Body.* New York: HarperCollins, 1991.

Donald Drake and Marian Uhlman — *Making Medicine, Making Money.* Kansas City, MO: Andrews & McMeel, 1993.

Steven R. Eastaugh — *Health Economics: Efficiency, Quality, and Equity.* Westport, CT: Auburn House, 1992.

Fred M. Frohock — *Healing Powers: Alternative Medicine, Spiritual Communities, and the State.* Chicago: University of Chicago Press, 1992.

John C. Goodman and Gerald L. Musgrave — *Patient Power: Solving America's Health Care Crisis.* Washington, DC: Cato Institute, 1992.

Iain Hay — *Money, Medicine, and Malpractice in American Society.* Westport, CT: Praeger, 1992.

Robert B. Helms, ed. — *American Health Policy: Critical Issues for Reform.* Washington, DC: The AEI Press, 1993.

Robert P. Huefner and Margaret P. Battin — *Changing to National Health Care: Ethical and Policy Issues.* Salt Lake City: University of Utah Press, 1992.

Institute of Medicine — *Assessing Health Care Reform.* Washington, DC: National Academy Press, 1993.

Stephen J. Isaacs and Ava C. Swartz — *The Consumer's Legal Guide to Today's Health Care: Your Medical Rights and How to Assert Them.* Boston: Houghton Mifflin, 1993.

Paul Jesilow, Henry N. Pontell, and Gilbert Geis — *Prescription for Profit: How Doctors Defraud Medicaid.* Berkeley: University of California Press, 1993.

Don W. Larson — *Medical Cost Crisis: A Common-Sense Solution.* Owatonna, MN: Bond Publishing Co., 1993.

Howard M. Leichter — *Health Policy Reform in America: Innovations from the States.* Armonk, NY: M.E. Sharpe, 1992.

Ruth Macklin — *Enemies of Patients.* New York: Oxford University Press, 1993.

Willard G. Manning et al., eds. — *The Costs of Poor Health Habits.* Cambridge, MA: Harvard University Press, 1991.

Michael Millman, ed. — *Access to Health Care in America.* Washington, DC: National Academy Press, 1993.

Miriam K. Mills and Robert H. Blank, eds. — *Health Insurance and Public Policy: Risk, Allocation, and Equity.* Westport, CT: Greenwood Press, 1993.

255

Bill Moyers	*Healing and the Mind*. New York: Doubleday/ Bantam, 1993.
Vicente Navarro	*Why the United States Does Not Have a National Health Program*. Amityville, NY: Baywood Publishing, 1992.
Mark V. Pauly, Patricia Danzon, Paul J. Feldstein, and John Hoff	*Responsible National Health Insurance*. Washington, DC: The AEI Press, 1992.
Lynn Payer	*Disease Mongers: How Doctors, Drug Companies, and Insurers Are Making You Feel Sick*. New York: Wiley, 1992.
Michael D. Reagan	*Curing the Crisis: Options for America's Health Care*. Boulder, CO: Westview Press, 1992.
Robert P. Rhodes	*Health Care Politics, Policy, and Distributive Justice: The Ironic Triumph*. Albany: State University of New York Press, 1992.
Marc A. Rodwin	*Medicine, Money, and Morals: Physicians' Conflicts of Interest*. New York: Oxford University Press, 1993.
Neil Rolde	*Your Money or Your Health: America's Cruel, Bureaucratic, and Horrendously Expensive Health Care System: How It Got That Way and What to Do About It!* New York: Paragon House, 1992.
C. Norman Shealy	*Third Party Rape: The Conspiracy to Rob You of Health Care*. St. Paul, MN: Galde Press, 1993.
Stephen M. Shortell and Uwe E. Reinhardt, eds.	*Improving Health Policy and Management: Nine Critical Issues for the 1990s*. Ann Arbor, MI: Health Administration Press, 1992.
F.A. Sloan, R.R. Bovbjerg, and P.B. Githens	*Insuring Medical Malpractice*. New York: Oxford University Press, 1991.
Martin A. Strosberg et al., eds.	*Rationing America's Health Care: The Oregon Plan and Beyond*. Washington, DC: The Brookings Institution, 1992.
Terree P. Wasley	*What Has Government Done to Our Health Care?* Washington, DC: Cato Institute, 1992.
Lawrence D. Weiss	*No Benefit: Crisis in America's Health Insurance Industry*. Boulder, CO: Westview Press, 1992.
John R. Wolfe	*The Coming Health Crisis: Who Will Pay for Care for the Aged in the 21st Century?* Chicago: University of Chicago Press, 1993.

Index

Health Insurance and Cost-
Containment Act, 223
health maintenance organizations
(HMOs)
health care rationing by, 240
managed competition and,
179-83, 240
physicians and, 80, 90, 91
Hentoff, Nat, 191
herbalism
effectiveness of, 97-100
should be integrated into
medicine, 107
high-risk behavior, 57
Himmelstein, David U., 134
Hoge, Nettie, 35
homeopathic medicine, 97-100,
115
hospitals
administrative costs of, 137-8
advertising and, 141
as greedy, 19, 31
emergency-room care in, 55
free care in, 221
length of patients' stay and, 28,
46, 51
lobbying and, 32
overabundance of, 66, 170
problems in, 79-80
relationships with doctors, 78,
79
hypnosis, 110, 114

imagery, 108, 110
immunizations, 97, 140, 172,
210, 234
infant mortality rates, 43, 56, 57,
158
Inlander, Charles B., 75
insurance, medical
costs of, 39
drug costs and, 214
employer-provided
as inadequate, 18
job-lock and, 73, 152-3
low-paying jobs and, 227
managed competition and,
179-80
mandatory provision is unjust,
36, 224-30
shifts costs to workers, 23, 34,
152-3
should be required, 218-23

small businesses and, 36, 135,
176, 179, 186, 219, 221-2, 229
government regulations inhibit,
148-9
inefficiency of, 40, 73
in other countries, 73
lack of, 55-6
malpractice awards and, 206,
207
managed competition and, 135,
137, 176-7
mandated-benefit laws, 23
people without
health care for, 54-5, 80, 221,
229
small business and, 179, 219
statistics on, 37, 55-6, 80, 143,
148, 152, 163, 221, 229, 232
pre-existing conditions and,
153, 180-1, 220, 222, 227
profits in, 137
public dissatisfaction with, 73
unemployment and, 19
women and, 220, 226-30
insurance companies
as greedy, 19, 233, 235
elimination of, 135
lobbying and, 32-7, 183
number of, 40
oppose reform, 34, 36, 183
Italy
dissatisfaction with health care
in, 73
health care spending in, 40
infant mortality rate in, 56
life expectancy in, 56

Jackson Hole Group, 175, 176
Japan
AIDS cases in, 57
doctors in, 60
health care costs in, 23, 34, 40,
170
health care system in, 60, 183
life expectancy in, 56, 57
Jecker, Nancy S., 224

Karp, Nathan, 17
Kemper, Vicki, 30
Krieger, Gary, 148

Lee, Robert W., 50
life expectancy

advocacy group), 36, 37
Purvis, Andrew, 120

quality of life
  health care rationing and, 194

Randal, Judith, 178
Rasell, Edie, 38
relaxation therapy, 108, 114
Relman, Arnold S., 65
Riggs, Webster, Jr., 55, 58
Robinson, David, 192, 193, 194
Rochefort, David A., 218
Royko, Mike, 81
Russia
  health care system in, 146
Ruttenberg, Joan E., 227

Schroeder, Steven A., 85
Schwartz, William B., 26
self-help groups, 109, 110, 114
Skocpol, Theda, 220
smoking
  health and, 47-50
social factors
  affect health care system,
    54-61, 82-3
socialism
  can solve health care problems,
    21
    con, 146-7
Social Security, 19, 51
Solovitch, Sara, 96
Spain
  infant mortality rate in, 56
sports medicine, 78, 118
Starr, Paul, 175
support groups, 109, 110, 114
surgery
  heart, 42, 59, 87, 110, 165, 171,
    174
  hernia, 58, 239
  unnecessary, 42, 78-9, 90
Sweden
  death rates in, 58
  health care spending in, 40, 167
  life expectancy in, 58
  malpractice system in, 141
Switzerland
  health care system in, 183
  life expectancy in, 58

Task Force on National Health
  Care Reform, 232

thalidomide, 211

uninsured persons
  health care for, 54-5, 80, 221,
    229
  public pays costs for, 221
  statistics on, 54-6, 80, 143, 148,
    152, 163, 232
unions
  insurance and, 226
United States
  Congress
    health care lobbying and,
      31-7, 183
    should adopt Canadian health
      care system, 151-9
      con, 160-8
    should nationalize health care,
      134-41
      con, 142-50, 177
Upjohn pharmaceutical
  company, 32, 210, 212

Van Deerlin, Lionel, 209
Veterans Administration
  health care and, 149-50
Victims of Chiropractic, 128-9

Wallis, Claudia, 108
Wassersug, Joseph D., 89, 103
Weidenbaum, Murray, 213
weight-loss clinics, 114, 140
Wiener, Joshua M., 187
Wofford, Harris, 35
Wolfe, Alan, 238
Wollstein, Jarret B., 142
women
  breast cancer and, 58, 109-10,
    176
  cesarian sections, 78, 237
  employer-provided insurance
    and, 220, 226-9
  Medicaid and, 227-8
  part-time employment and,
    220, 226-7
  physicians take advantage of,
    78
  self-care and, 109
  Woolhandler, Steffie, 134

X rays
  chiropractors and, 121, 130
  new technology and, 27
  overuse of, 41, 233